Chiropractic

Chiropractic: A Philosophy for Alternative Health Care

Ian D. Coulter, PhD

Health Consultant, RAND, Santa Monica, California
Professor, School of Dentistry, University of California, Los Angeles
Professor, Los Angeles College of Chiropractic

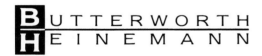

OXFORD   AUCKLAND   BOSTON   JOHANNESBURG   MELBOURNE   NEW DELHI

Butterworth-Heinemann
Linacre House, Jordan Hill, Oxford OX2 8DP
225 Wildwood Avenue, Woburn, MA 01801–2041
A division of Reed Educational and Professional Publishing Ltd

A member of the Reed Elsevier plc group

First published 1999
Reprinted 2001

British Library Cataloguing in Publication Data
A catalogue record for this book is available from the British Library

Library of Congress Cataloging in Publication Data
A catalogue record for this book is available from the Library of Congress

ISBN 0 7506 4006 5

Composition by Genesis Typesetting, Laser Quay, Rochester, Kent
Printed and bound in Great Britain by
Biddles Ltd, *www.biddles.co.uk*

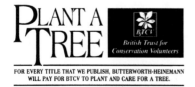

I shall be telling this with a sigh
Somewhere ages and ages hence
Two roads diverged in a wood, and I
I took the one less travelled by
And that has made all the difference

The Road Not Taken Robert Frost

I dedicate this book to Dr Douglas Brown, who set me on the road less travelled and stayed to see the journey through.

Contents

Foreword – Chiropractic: the return of philosophy to medicine?

Wayne B. Jonas

Chiropractic medicine is an important and growing part of our culture[1]. Therefore, knowing about chiropractic medicine is increasingly important for physicians, researchers, those in health care policy and the public. There are now two books to help those who wish to understand chiropractic more and, in combination, they provide a detailed and comprehensive overview of the profession. These are the report on Chiropractic Medicine in the United States by Daniel Cherkin *et al.* published by the Agency for Health Care Policy and Research, and this book by Ian Coulter[2]. These two books are a great match because whilst the former is comprehensive, Dr Coulter goes into depth. Dr Coulter, a longtime student and researcher of chiropractic, has provided us with an exposé of the chiropractic profession and its relationship to both conventional medicine and other alternative medicine practices. In addition, he has placed this within a historical, practice and philosophical context like no one else can. This book is not only an education about chiropractic, but a critique of conventional medicine and the newly resurgent complementary and alternative medicine.

I am often asked if chiropractic medicine can be investigated using conventional scientific methods (such as blinded randomized controlled trials). My standard response to this is that not only can these methods be used but they *must* be used. Modern scientific methodology is constructed to separate belief and magic from objective observations by using theory and experiment. This has not always been the case in medicine and is not so even now for some areas. However, conventional medicine at least has continued to emphasize science as a basis for its practice. Many terrible treatments have been eliminated as scientific and evidence-based medicine evolved. But the progress of science into medicine has not been without resistance. Until recently, most medical procedures were adopted because of power or profit rather than evidence[3]. Eventually, however, a medicine based on laboratory methods, the clinical trial, and theories derived from these has emerged.

The struggle to incorporate more science into medicine has provided us with methodological tools to help separate belief from actuality[4]. One has to use good methods – it is better to have no facts than false facts; this is because it is harder to find true answers in a sea of falsity. Often we spend generations unlearning the false before we can look for the true. Yet, even in the midst of these developments there have always been waves of interest in holistic medicine as an alternative perspective to a materialistic and reductionist biomedicine. Between 1920–50, for example, a rising interest in holism and a reaction against laboratory medicine was quite prominent[5]. However, this movement largely died out after World War II. Chiropractic, since it remained outside and often in conflict with conventional medicine, was able to hold onto a holistic philosophy. Dr Coulter elegantly outlines how this is achieved and also where chiropractic fails to operate holistically.

If chiropractic is to be legitimized in terms of modern science what will be required? A characteristic of modern science is that it is theory driven. This does not mean just any theory, but theory that uses a specific language and logic. The language is one of materialism and objectivity in which measurement is possible and reproducible. The logic is one of testing; and experimentation, which assumes that linear causation and probability exist and can be demonstrated. Proof and especially dis-proof are paramount in modern science. Thus, a theory should be able to predict observations that can be disproven and then produce revision of theory and guidance for future testing. Empirical testing without such a theory is generally considered futile.

There is still considerable controversy within the chiropractic profession itself over the value and nature of its foundations and philosophy. Vitalism, holism, naturalism, therapeutic conservatism and critical rationalism are not in themselves a distinguishing feature of chiropractic alone. Some of these concepts lead to theories that are incompatible with current biomedical assumptions. Should chiro-practic link itself to accepted theories in biomedicine (an approach that would likely gain credibility) or should it seek to validate the theoretical implications of its own philosophy at the risk of continued marginalization? The latter is, while risky, more likely to preserve chiropractic identity in the face of rapid globalization of health care concepts.

Chiropractic now faces a dilemma and has to choose how it will develop its philosophy and science in the future. For example, there is no accepted evidence that spinal realignment is the basis for the observed changes after chiropractic treatment and the vitalist issue has been bypassed in the West since no convincing demonstration of purported 'subtle energy' exists. What if no model for the validation of spinal manipulation is discovered, no animal model to study its mechanisms is developed, and no objective demonstration of replicable and cost-effective manipulation-based diagnosis and treatment can be shown in clinical trials? What if these most fundamental parameters for the proof of chiropractic medicine are not forthcoming? Would we then recommend that chiropractic be used less, identifying it only as an elaborate and long-term placebo effect? Would chiropractic research then change to focus on why people actually seek chiropractic care and the benefits received? Coulter shows us that patients often seek and receive non-manipulative aspects of chiropractic care, such as the reception of health education, counselling, and the time spent with the practitioner. In addition, patients often get satisfaction from some meaning in their illness derived from explanations by the chiropractor about why they are suffering and the options they have to alleviate that suffering. These are not unique to chiropractic, however. Will a philosophy of chiropractic emerge that can generate its own testable theories and models that set it apart from other health care practices but do not depend on spinal subluxation? Dr Coulter has laid the foundation for the development of such a philosophy and so, perhaps, for a theory that can allow chiropractic to enter into the scientific age without losing its identity.

What then should we do about chiropractic research? It is certainly unreasonable to ignore chiropractic research, as has been done by both the chiropractic profession and conventional medicine until recently. On the other hand, it is of marginal use to simply accumulate random anomalous findings around subluxation and energy flow, if they have no theoretical grounding in modern scientific language and concepts. Even if chiropractic should discover acceptable mechanisms for explaining spinal manipulation the profession risks becoming legitimized in a way that could marginalize the patients for whom chiropractic care is important – those who are seeking out a more person-oriented approach than conventional medicine frequently offers. Thus, health services research and research on the social dynamics of the practitioner–patient interaction should not be neglected. Finally, Dr Coulter makes it clear that simply looking for a major 'homerun' experiment showing that chiropractic either works or does not work, is also not likely to be useful. Clinical research is not so sensitive as to prove or disprove the value of any complex practice with only a few clinical trials. Only a systematic program can do this.

A philosophy and science of chiropractic can be developed but will require the kind of deep and insightful self-criticism that Dr Coulter supplies. The challenge to chiropractic is to use its philosophy and research to go beyond simply the establishment and propagation of the profession. It will require a scholarly agenda that explores not only the reality of chiropractic procedures, but also their utility. It must examine not only the effectiveness of chiropractic practices, but also its overall value to the health care system. If this happens, then surely Dr Coulter is right in pointing to chiropractic as an exemplar for all complementary medicine. Indeed, the return of philosophy to science can help us reformulate the role that science will play in the global medicine of the next millennium[6].

References

[1] Eisenberg, D. M., Davis, R.B., Ettner S, *et al.* (1998). Trends in alternative medicine use in the United States 1990–1997: Results of a follow-up national survey. *JAMA*, **280**,1569–1575.

[2] Cherkin, D.C., Mootz, R.D. (1997). *Chiropractic in the United States: Training, Practice and Research*. Agency for Health Care Policy and Research.

[3] McKinlay, J.B. (1981). From 'promising report' to 'standard procedure': Seven stages in the career of a medical innovation. *Milbank Memorial Fund Quarterly/Health and Society*, **59**:374–411.

[4] Jonas, W.B. (1997). Clinical trials for chronic disease: randomized, controlled clinical trials are essential. *J. NIH Research*, **9**:33–9.

[5] Lawrence, C. and Weisz, G. (1998). *Greater Than the Parts. Holism in Biomedicine, 1920–1950*. Oxford University Press.

[6] Linde, K., Jonas, W.B. (1999) Evaluating complementary and alternative medicine: The balance of rigor and relevance. In: *Essentials of Complementary and Alternative Medicine* (W. B. Jonas and J. S. Levin, eds), pp.57–71. Lipincott Williams and Wilkins.

Preface

In an era when there is rapidly increasing interest in, and use of, complementary and alternative health care (CAM) and its newer appellation, integrative medicine, chiropractic provides an exemplar of how a particular philosophy of health, and a particular practice of health care, was kept alive in the face of unremitting opposition from mainstream medicine. Chiropractors, and the other non-mainstream health providers, have maintained a perspective that increasingly resonates well with contemporary thought about health and well-being. They have kept alive the clinical art of chiropractic, and an art that contemporary medicine has lost and could relearn from chiropractors. While there is considerable debate about the extent to which these practices were 'alternative' and the extent to which they have become mainstream (in the sense that will be made clear in this book), they were clearly a different way of thinking about health, health care, the role of the health-care provider and the health encounter. Furthermore, they now provide a rich source for developing contemporary concepts about health.

However, the chiropractic health encounter poses a puzzle. While it is clear that the patients experience chiropractic as unique, and different to the medical encounter, it is not quite so obvious why. The health conditions treated by chiropractic are not unique; they can be found equally in medical offices. The major form of therapy is also not unique – manipulation can be found in physical therapy, osteopathy, naturopathy and manual medicine, to name but a few. The patient's perception of a unique chiropractic experience, however, led this author to a 20-year exploration. This book continues that exploration, and investigates the extent to which a combination of a philosophy of health and health care and a set of treatment practices (the clinical art of chiropractic) creates a constellation that is uniquely chiropractic.

The exploration combines extensive empirical research on chiropractic, but is guided by sociological and philosophical concepts. Chapter 1 begins by focusing on what chiropractors call *chiropractic philosophy*, but which (for reasons developed in the chapter) will be called, in this work, the philosophy of chiropractic. In attempting to develop a model of the health encounter found in chiropractic, and a model of the education of chiropractors, it is necessary to turn to philosophy and the concept developed by Thomas Kuhn: paradigms. Since the concept is much broader than theory or models, and allows for the inclusion of beliefs, values, language, concepts, puzzles, research traditions and metaphysical elements, it allows investigation of the full complexity of chiropractic. The chiropractic paradigm is explored in Chapter 2.

A key part of the chiropractic paradigm, and one which has split the profession historically into two camps, is the metaphysical belief system known as *vitalism*. Within philosophy, vitalism has generally been portrayed as a failed metaphysic. This is somewhat unfortunate, because it is an underpinning *a priori* construct for virtually all the alternative health-care paradigms, and for holistic medicine. Once again, it will be philosophy that provides the understanding for what vitalism involves and its influence on the chiropractic paradigm. This work is contained in Chapter 3.

From the work on paradigms and metaphysics, it is then possible to attempt a reformulation of a philosophy of chiropractic as opposed to chiropractic philosophy (Chapter 4). Chiropractic combines five distinct philosophies: vitalism, holism, naturalism, therapeutic conservatism and critical rationalism. These in turn give rise to a particular conception of health, and a particular form of health care. It also provides a distinct concept of the role of the health-care provider or healer. Ultimately, all these matters of philosophy have substantive importance only if they make a difference in the delivery of health care – that is, a difference in the health-care encounter. Therefore, Chapter 5 examines the research on the chiropractic health encounter. It shows that the distinct health encounter arises from and is understandable in terms of the philosophical concepts. It is here that we can begin to understand what chiropractic, along with other alternative paradigms, has to offer contemporary health care. Partly because of its isolation and the hostility from medicine, chiropractic has been free to preserve an alternative way of thinking about health and health care and, within its own educational institutions, to embrace a variety of philosophical positions. To this extent, chiropractic and the other alternative disciplines have preserved a concept of health that dates back to the ancient Greeks.

In the final chapter, Chapter 6, we will examine the history of medicine and chiropractic in this century. Chiropractic arose as a reaction to medicine, and most of its history has been characterized by unremitting hostility between the two professions. From these two separate histories two distinct health encounters arose, and these are compared and contrasted. The chapter closes with some thought about the future of chiropractic.

In summary, like many of the alternative health-care paradigms, chiropractic is a sociological enigma. Confronted with extensive hostility and conflict from medicine, and a well-orchestrated attempt to eradicate it as a health profession, it has not only survived but has flourished. In North America, the population using chiropractic has doubled in the past 20 years. The number of chiropractors tripled from 1970 to 1990, and will double again by 2010, during which time medical practitioners will increase by only 16 per cent[1]. In Western society it is the most firmly entrenched, and the most frequently used, of the alternative providers, and this leads us to the inevitable conclusion that it is meeting some fundamental health, social and/ or psychological need. Its success alone warrants sociological attention.

The intellectual journey over the past 20 years has led the author to the conclusion that chiropractic and, by implication, the alternative health-care providers, do provide a different philosophical way of conceptualizing health and illness. It is a philosophy that leads to a distinct way of interacting with the patient and of thinking about outcomes. Given the rather wholesale retreat of medicine from philosophy in the twentieth century, this perspective has largely been preserved as a living philosophy by the alternative providers. While it was a perspective that characterized medicine for much of its early history, and survives in areas such as holistic medicine, its loss had serious consequences for health care.

Health has not generally been viewed as a proper object of philosophical study. It is not well known that health and health care were important topics for Plato and Aristotle, as well as for

Descartes, Locke and Kant. Few people know that the dominant school of medicine in Europe until the seventeenth century – Galenic medicine – was an application of central themes in Aristotle's natural philosophy, or that many of the schools that followed were highly influenced by Descartes' philosophy of man. Even fewer would believe that philosophical analysis or speculation could make any valuable contribution to modern medicine. Medicine has for a long time – so many would put it – been liberating itself from the bonds of philosophy in its move to become an empirical science.

Nordenfelt[2]

The position taken in this book is that, at the end of the twentieth century, where major diseases are related to lifestyle and have largely been unresponsive to treatment within the reductionistic, biomedical paradigm, there is an important place for the alternative philosophies. The philosophy of chiropractic in this context provides an interesting exemplar for all alternative health care.

References

[1] Cooper, R. A. and Stoflet, S. J. (1993). Trends in the education and practice of alternative medicine. *Health Affairs*, **15,** 226–38.
[2] Nordenfelt, L. (1987). *On the Nature of Health*. D. Reidel.

<table>
<tr><td>CHAPTER
1</td><td># Chiropractic philosophy has no future</td></tr>
</table>

Although chiropractic philosophy is widely talked about within the profession, and taught within chiropractic institutions and continuing education programmes, it is, in fact, a misnomer[1]. What is referred to as chiropractic philosophy is frequently not philosophy at all or, where it is, it can clearly be shown not to be uniquely, or even originally, chiropractic[2].

To understand this point it is necessary to have some notion of what constitutes philosophy – philosophy as an activity and not some body of doctrine[3]. What chiropractors call chiropractic philosophy most closely resembles doctrine or dogma. Simply put, the purpose of philosophical activity is clarification of thought. It is reflective activity that leads to clarification of thought:

> As such it has no subject matter of its own; it consists, instead, of critical reflections on other subjects, that is, of philosophizing about other subjects.
>
> Ladd[4]

Hence we find such areas as the philosophy *of* law, the philosophy *of* education, the philosophy *of* science, the philosophy *of* art, and so on. These areas do not speak of themselves as philosophy, and to do so would be to make a fairly arrogant claim. Historically, and currently in some instances, chiropractic describes itself as the philosophy, science and art of things natural. But what could such a statement mean? The science of all things natural? Chiropractic is hardly that. The science of some things natural? Hardly that either. Perhaps the science of a few things natural pertaining to health? Of course, the broader question is whether it is even a science to begin with. Similarly with its claim to be the philosophy of things natural. This is not a distinction that would make much sense to a philosopher; nor would it describe any field that would be recognized as a branch of philosophy.

Ladd[4] proposes four propositions to capture the essence of philosophy:

1   Philosophy may be thought of as the philosophy of something

2   Philosophy is inevitably critical, and necessarily implies a critical evaluation of the concepts and the structures in which they are framed

3   Philosophy is problem-oriented

4   Philosophy is inexorably controversial.

For the most part, what passes for chiropractic philosophy lacks any critical evaluation and amounts to little more than the reiteration of principles and metaphysical statements either made by the founding fathers, or thought to be crucial by chiropractic writers. In sociological terms, it more resembles justifications for chiropractic, and what sociologists would term the role ideology. The method by which philosophy achieves a critical perspective is through conceptual analysis.

In addition to the four propositions, philosophy also consists of branches that have been established to assist in conceptual analysis and that form sub-disciplines. These include the following:

❑ Ontology – which deals with questions of the ultimate nature of reality
❑ Epistemology – which deals with how we know, the theories about knowledge itself
❑ Aesthetics – which deals with questions of beauty
❑ Ethics – which deals with questions of right and wrong
❑ Logic – which deals with principles of correct or reliable inference.

To claim that there is a chiropractic philosophy is to claim that chiropractic has developed a new and unique branch of philosophy, and this can hardly be substantiated. Nor is it likely that this is what chiropractors have meant[5].

It is possible to argue that this distinction between a philosophy of chiropractic and chiropractic philosophy is simple a semantic quibble. Unfortunately, it has had consequences for chiropractic way beyond those of simple semantics. For those knowledgeable about philosophy it has made chiropractic look philosophically ignorant, and has perhaps prevented more philosophers taking an active interest in this branch of the healing arts. In this way, chiropractic has not been strengthened by the baptism of intellectual critique provided by independent scholars in philosophy. Within the profession itself, this lack of understanding of philosophy has prevented the development of a self-critical tradition in which the philosophical concepts could be developed, enriched, rejected, modified and added to. Those who did critique the philosophical ideas of D. D. and B. J. Palmer were labelled heretics, and chiropractic has been split for the last 100 years into at least two metaphysical camps because of the inability to have honest, intellectual and critical debate over philosophical issues. In America the groups remain split politically, despite extensive efforts during the last 10 years to come to some reconciliation. The damage this has done to the profession externally and politically is difficult to determine, but a house divided against itself clearly expends much of its effort, and a considerable part of its resources, on fighting internal battles. Even worse, the descriptions of chiropractic – such as the philosophy, science and art of things natural – were presented to the public and legislators as serious definitions. That they had great difficulty in understanding what chiropractic distinguished is evidenced by the incredible variety of chiropractic Acts that were enacted by the various legislators and jurisdictions. In Canada, for example, historically no two provinces within the same nation enacted the same definition of chiropractic.

The chiropractic 100-year war

Although the full metaphysical nature of the doctrinal split within the chiropractic profession will be discussed in Chapter 3, it is necessary here to give a brief outline of what the split was about[6]. Chiropractic has been characterized by two very broad metaphysical camps. One of these subscribes to the initial concepts of D. D. Palmer, which held that the body was subject to both an innate and a universal intelligence. This camp can be termed the *innatists*. Metaphysically speaking, this is a belief in vitalism. The other camp is distinguished mainly by its rejection of both innate and universal intelligence, and will be termed here the *rationalists*. For the most part, this group turned to the basic biological sciences upon which to found a 'chiropractic philosophy'. Part of the conflict arose because of D. D. Palmer's own confusion about philosophy and its role[7]. Furthermore, very early in chiropractic history, so-called 'chiropractic philosophy' became a legal stratagem for defending the profession rather than an exercise to clarify the nature of chiropractic[8].

Within chiropractic, the conflict between the two camps had an immediate impact on practice, and resulted in two types of chiropractors. The so-called *straights* claimed to hold true to the original 'chiropractic philosophy', and practised spine only, hands only chiropractic – that is, they used only their hands and manipulated only the spine. The counter-group, known in chiropractic as *mixers*, embraced a much broader paradigm, using an array of adjunctive therapies (heat, electrical, water, supplements etc.) and embracing a much wider scope of practice (at the very least, treating all the articulated joint structures of the body and not just the spine).

At the heart of the split was the concept of innate. This is a metaphysical construct, an ontological statement about the ultimate nature of the world (universal intelligence) and of the human body (innate intelligence). Briefly, it postulates that the universe is the reflection of an intelligent life force, and that this life force finds its expression in the human body through innate intelligence.

Innate intelligence is captured in the concept *vis medicatrix naturae*, the innate tendency of the body to heal itself. The notion of the innate is clearly an *a priori* assumption that cannot be subjected to testing. For the rationalists, it is a semi-religious concept that has no place in a discipline portraying itself as a science. For them, it persists simply as a dogma.

Conclusion

In conclusion, what has been termed chiropractic philosophy for the most part does not meet the generally accepted criteria of what constitutes philosophy. This confusion has caused both dissension within chiropractic itself, and an external rejection of a philosophy of chiropractic as a serious discourse worthy of the attention of scholars. A philosophy of chiropractic would on the one hand lead to a fuller understanding of chiropractic, and on the other to a critical advancement of the central concepts of the profession. It would also serve as an exemplar of a philosophy of alternative health care.

References

[1] Weiant, C. W. (1981). Chiropractic philosophy. The misnomer that plagues the profession. *Arch Calif. Chiropr. Assoc.*, **5**, 15–22.
[2] Coulter, I. D. (1991). Chiropractic philosophy has no future. *Chiropr. J. Aust.*, **21**, 129–31.
[3] Wittgenstein, L. (1961). *Tractatus Logico-Philosophicus* (translated by D. F. Pers and B. F. McGuiness). Routledge, Kegan Paul.
[4] Ladd, J. (1979). Philosophy of medicine. In *Changing Values in Medicine* (E. J. Cassell and M. Sigler, eds), pp. 205–16. University Publishers of America.
[5] Coulter, I. D. (1992). Uses and abuses of philosophy in chiropractic. *Philosoph. Constr. Chiropr. Prof.*, **2(1)**, 3–7.
[6] Coulter, I. D. (1989). The chiropractic wars, or the enemy within. *Am. J. Chiropr. Med.*, **2(2)**, 64–6.
[7] Donahue, J. D. (1986). D. D. Palmer and innate intelligence: development, division and derision. *Chiropr. Hist.*, **6**, 31–6.
[8] Donahue, J. D. (1994). Metaphysics, rationality and science. *J. Manipul. Physiol. Ther.*, **17(1)**, 54–5.

The chiropractic paradigm

In 1962, Thomas Kuhn published *The Structure of Scientific Revolutions*[1], in which he introduced the concept of paradigms to describe the broad conceptual frameworks shared by scientists and that guided their work even prior to the existence of a common theory. Kuhn's initial problem was how to account for something that a community of scientists shared, and that allowed them to solve puzzles and have unanimity in choosing problems and judging solutions, when there was no common theory as such. To understand chiropractic as a paradigm, it is first necessary to understand Kuhn's concept of paradigm.

Kuhn's paradigms

Kuhn derived his notion of paradigms from his work on the history of science[2]. Historically, science had been portrayed as a rational accumulation of increasingly truer theories and information. It was seen as steadily accumulative, integrative and logical. Kuhn's own work found science to proceed in a way analogous to art, and with what he termed *gestalt transformations* – for example, one day scientists subscribe to a belief in absolute time and space (pre-Einstein), and the next they subscribe to a belief in relative time and space (post-Einstein). Such a drastic change in perception is a gestalt transformation. The term gestalt transformation comes from the psychology of perception, where certain objects can be seen as one thing or another but not the two simultaneously (the classic example is a figure that can be seen either as a vase or as two faces). The mind cannot entertain the two images simultaneously. Kuhn's conclusion was that the history of science was in fact a distorted history, a reconstruction that made the history of science appear more rational than it actually was.

Normal science

Kuhn identified two distinct periods in science; normal and revolution. In the period of normal science, an area or specialty (and, in some rare instances, most of science) is dominated by a paradigm. The paradigm may include theory or predate it, but also covers a wide range of beliefs, values and even techniques of research. However, the essential feature is that it provides the frame of reference within which the science proceeds. It provides the questions thought to be worth pursuing, and the criteria for judging whether answers have been found. During periods of normal science, the activity of scientists is not concerned with confirming or falsifying the basic premises of the paradigm (that is, the work is not about testing the paradigm), but with applying it over as wide a field as possible. To distinguish the nature of normal science, Kuhn used the concept of puzzle solving as opposed to problem solving.

The essential feature of a puzzle is that a solution exists within the terms of the puzzle, and the challenge is to find the solution. A problem, on the other hand, may not be solvable by the paradigm. Furthermore, with a puzzle there is agreement about what constitutes a solution. In a jigsaw puzzle, you cannot reshape the pieces to make them fit; each piece has one location only, but you do know that a location exists and the objective is to find it. A puzzle is seen as a test of the ingenuity of the researcher, and failure to solve the puzzle is not seen as a test of the paradigm but as a test of the scientist. Puzzle solving, however, can only occur after the paradigm has reached a certain level of maturity, since it involves some concrete predictions for a range of phenomena. Of course scientists can ignore engaging in the puzzles and attempt to test the paradigm, but this will not result in a period of normal science.

Initially, Kuhn conceived such paradigms as a form of dogma subscribed to by the scientists. Periods of normal science, while very productive, are restrictive. Instead of the view of science progressing on a broad front, Kuhn's work suggested that normal science involved very focused efforts on accepted puzzles. It is during normal science that we get the sequential development usually portrayed for all science. However, since no paradigm can solve all the puzzles, with the passage of time the paradigm accumulates anomalies. Such anomalies are anomalies only for the paradigm, but they will not automatically lead to the overthrow of the paradigm, even when they seem to constitute a falsification of the paradigm itself. They eventually result in a crisis for the paradigm, and lead to competing paradigms. Such competitors involve a gestalt trans-formation and, in a sense, cannot be compared directly to the existing paradigm – they are incommensurable. As with the figures described above, the vase and the faces, they cannot both be maintained simultaneously. Kuhn was also unique in arguing that the decision to abandon one paradigm and convert to another was not based on logical grounds (on scientific evidence). Where commitment to the first paradigm is an act of faith, moving to a new paradigm involves an act of conversion.

Disciplinary matrix

In his later work, Kuhn[3] used the concept of *disciplinary matrix* to capture the full extent of a paradigm. This includes the symbolic generalizations, shared models and values, language, shared techni-cal achievements and concrete solutions to puzzles that he termed exemplars, etc. An example of a paradigm would be Euclidian geometry. It is based on an *a priori* assumption that two parallel lines do not meet and if, but only if, that is true, the rest of Euclidian geometry is true. However, Euclidian geometry cannot establish the truth of the original premise. The system is deduc-tively true, but only if the *a priori* postulate is. The way in which Euclidian geometry was traditionally taught is an example of Kuhn's exemplars. Students were given puzzles to solve within the paradigm, such as proving the theorem of Pythagorus. They were also taught by learning theorems that had already been solved (exemplars), so that they could apply these in new situations thought to be similar. They came to solve problems in geometry in a Euclidian way.

Development of a new paradigm

A new paradigm may be the work of a single individual, often young and frequently marginal, but unless it converts others, it will not flourish. It is successful only in the extent to which it converts others and they in turn attract followers. Kuhn was also unique in arguing the new paradigm is not necessarily truer than the older paradigm, only that it was different. Masterman[4], while isolating at least 21 different uses of the word paradigm by Kuhn, has identified three major types of paradigms; metaphysical paradigms; sociological paradigms and construct paradigms. The metaphysical paradigm refers to the beliefs, myths and new ways of seeing things that accompany paradigms, and this would include the philosophical presuppositions of the paradigm. The sociological paradigm is the recognizable, identifiable social group embracing the paradigm. Here, actual scientists behave in similar fashion even though they have no shared theory. A construct paradigm occurs when something such as instrumentation or textbook examples gives rise to a paradigm. Kuhn's theory is directed to the formative stages of the development of science. If scientists behave similarly without a theory, it must be through shared values and beliefs and an already established set of practices. However, this presupposes that the scientists know they are following a paradigm. The primary sense of a paradigm must therefore be a philosophical one. To discover this, Kuhn felt that we need to examine the original 'trick' (which may be technology, a mathematical formula, etc.), coupled with the insight that this is applicable to a field that establishes a set of habits, a sociological paradigm. From this original trick will develop all the experimental procedures, mathematical formulations and work that will constitute the scientific achievement of the paradigm. All the metaphysics, philosophy, theories, techniques, research and puzzle solving may also develop from this trick, along with the social organization of the scientists.

Extent of a paradigm

A paradigm may be shared over a whole discipline or within sub-fields and, on occasions, over the whole of science (for example, Darwin's theory of evolution). The size of the community embraced by the paradigm may also vary considerably. Several paradigms may exist in a field simultaneously, but the dominant conflict will usually be between two competing paradigms. Scientists are socialized into the paradigms, not by a formal introduction to a set of rules, but much in the same way as a child learns to speak a language without knowing any of the rules of grammar. This is a process of ostension. By doing Euclidian puzzles, the student comes to see new puzzles in a Euclidian way and will attempt to solve them within that framework. In calculating the surface area of a cone, we come to see it as the equivalent of a stack of a series of small disks. By doing the exemplars we internalize the norms, without being able to articulate the norms or rules. This is a process of learning quite distinct from learning through replication by rules. A child is not taught to recognize a duck by learning the sufficient and necessary conditions of classifying something as a duck, but by being shown a picture or a real duck and being taught the word. By applying the word over a range of animals and being corrected, a child comes to identify a duck correctly, but may never be able to give the rules for doing so. Children use language correctly, and can correct adults in their speech, and yet do not know the rules of grammar and syntax. If they learn them at all, it is after they can actually use language. Newtonian scientists will therefore think and act in a Newtonian paradigm, even if they cannot clearly delineate the features of the paradigm.

Implications of Kuhn's theory

The implications of Kuhn's theory for science are problematic for scientists. If scientific research is paradigm-bounded – that is, the paradigm defines the puzzles and what is an acceptable answer, gives the language and concepts to frame the work and provides the technology, mathematical formulas, etc. – then the existence of an objective science becomes questionable. Evidence is relative to a particular paradigm. Furthermore, since concepts are defined within the terms of the paradigm, differing paradigms (even where they use the same concepts) cannot be compared – they are incommensurable. For example, while Newton's and Einstein's paradigms may use the same concepts, because the *a priori* assumptions of the two paradigms are incompatible (either space and time are absolute *or* they are relative; they cannot be both), we cannot use one paradigm to knock the other out. In terms of formal logic, commensurability demands invariance in the meaning of the terms. If the terms between paradigms are not held to have constant meanings, then you are comparing apples and oranges. If the two paradigms are truly incommensurable, no comparisons are possible between them – including the notion that one is a scientific advancement over the other.

There is however a further problem, that of comparability. Not only can you not strictly compare the competing paradigms, but you cannot use an experiment in nature to decide the issue. Since any such comparison must be done within the terms of reference of the paradigm, nature itself cannot be approached directly. Kuhn therefore undermined two of the fundamental tenets of an objectivist philosophy of science; commensurability and comparability. Kuhn has argued that the paradigms are not completely incommensurable, but that the problem is one of translating one language into another. It can be done, but you cannot get a complete translation and some things will not translate at all (often humour falls into this category). There exists no neutral language for translation.

Conclusion

The notions of scientists indulging in acts of faith, converting, and subscribing to dogma did not endear Kuhn to scientists, historians or many philosophers. His account of science posed a radical challenge to the traditional view, and undermined its objectivist claim to produce independent data. Although there has been considerable criticism of Kuhn's work, many of his critics have been forced to develop concepts that are not all that dissimilar. In summary, Kuhn's work established that previous historical accounts of science were inadequate; that scientists seem to act with the same types of irrationality as others, subject to dogma, faith, conversions, revolutions, and gestalt switches; that science was not just a system of continuous revolution and falsification but consisted of periods of normal science; and that this not only occurred, but was constructive for science.

On a superficial level, Kuhn's theory would appear to capture much of chiropractic history very well; the dogmaticism and irrationality, the role of metaphysical paradigms, conversions, faith, the inability of chiropractors to articulate their paradigm clearly, and the competing gestalts. Chiropractic would seem to offer a fertile field to examine the ideas of Kuhn.

The chiropractic paradigm of D. D. Palmer

In the history of chiropractic, the founding of the profession occurred in 1895 when D. D. Palmer restored hearing to a deaf person by manipulating his spine. While this incident has been ridiculed by opponents of chiropractic, and its historical veracity challenged even within the profession (including the date of the event), it is interesting to note that the incident has all the characteristics of a construct paradigm – that is, a trick that led to a metaphysical approach to health. Palmer later claimed that there was nothing accidental or crude about this adjustment, but that it was specific and was carried out with a full expectation of the outcome because it was a manifestation of an already thought out theory. Some writers have questioned whether Palmer simply indulged in hindsight and may not have been all that certain of what he had discovered at the time. However, it is after this event that chiropractic was articulated as a paradigm with its own teaching institutions and practices; that is, it became a sociological paradigm. Furthermore, it is only after this incident that the metaphysical paradigm based on the notions of universal and innate intelligence was developed. D. D. Palmer's definition of chiropractic was the philosophy, science and art of things natural; a system of adjusting articulations of the spinal column, by hand only, for the correction of the cause of disease.

Prior to his establishment of chiropractic, Palmer had practised as a magnetic healer. His involvement in such areas as spiritualism and theosophy has been documented, as well as his knowledge of the metaphysical movement[5]. Palmer had been treating people for problems related to nerves (inflammation), and had been puzzled by the fact that some were afflicted by illness while others were not while sharing the same environment. The theory of illness embraced by the paradigm is fundamentally a neural theory. In simple terms, an intact nervous system is essential for the body to maintain health. Disruption to the nervous system results in dis-ease (as opposed to disease). One such disruption could be impairment of the nerves in the spinal column through misalignment of the vertebra, termed a subluxation. If this is removed through manipulation, the nerves are restored to their normal function. Palmer believed that the nervous system holds the major co-ordination function of the body, and the seat of the system is not the brain but the spinal column. From here, nerves run to all the organs of the body through the foramen of the vertebra. Palmer's theory has been portrayed historically as a 'pinched nerve' theory, although this is an over-simplification of his ideas.

The metaphysical and philosophical paradigm

In addition to the theoretical elements (e.g. the subluxation theory), a metaphysical paradigm also emerged. This is found in the onto-logical propositions formulated by both D. D. Palmer and his son, B. J. Palmer, which are assumptions about the nature of the universe and the body. In this paradigm, as opposed to that of medicine, the cause of disease is not to be found outside the body but within. Where the germ theory of disease sees a body invaded by germs from the outside, the chiropractic belief was that, as long as the body is functioning normally, it is able to combat disease naturally. This is a metaphysical belief that postulates that the body can heal itself through a life force called, in this instance, innate intelligence (or just innate). D. D. Palmer considered this force to be responsible for the vitality of the body. His metaphysical paradigm is just one expression of a much broader metaphysical belief called vitalism that was shared by most of the alternative health providers in the nineteenth century. The essential features of innate are that we are born with it, it controls all the functions of the body, and it is expressed through the nervous system. However, innate is part of universal intelligence (basically, it is the bodily expression of universal intelligence). The concept of universal intelligence simply acknowledges that the universe was created by a universal intelligence. While the brain is the seat of innate intelligence, it is the nervous system that acts as the communication system that informs innate about the state of the body. Innate intelligence is the product of evolution, and retains all the knowledge of eternity with regard to the body[6].

Palmer's philosophy of health

D. D. Palmer's metaphysical paradigm involves *a priori* presuppositions that are ontological in nature but also result in a theoretical commitment. As *a priori*, they are taken for granted presuppositions whose truth or falsity is not challenged. Such presuppositions are empirically unverifiable views. Palmer's philosophy of health is derivable from his metaphysical beliefs. The concept of innate presupposes the notion that the total body is an integrated system that functions holistically. As long as it retains its integrity, the body's natural tendency is toward health. Chiropractic does not therefore, in a strict sense, treat disease; it treats the body to enable it to continue to combat disease itself. The paradigm distinguishes between symptoms and causes of disease. Diseases, as they are commonly conceived, are symptoms in this paradigm. It is for this reason that chiropractic historically distinguished disease from dis-ease. The latter refers to a lack of ease on the part of innate, which leads to an inability of the body to heal itself. This position did not deny that micro-organisms were important, and the early chiropractic programmes all taught hygiene – which would not make much sense if chiropractors had rejected the germ theory of disease outright. What they had rejected was the dominance of the germ theory. They held, as did most of the alternative paradigms, that the germ theory of disease could not explain the distribution of disease – why is it that not everyone in the same bacterially dangerous environment comes down with the illness? Micro-organisms, in this view, are a stimulating factor, but tissue resistance (or lack of it) is the predisposing factor for disease. Palmer's view was that, by fighting the micro-organism, traditional medicine combats only the symptoms and not the cause of disease.

'Naturalness'

Related to the belief in the body's natural ability and tendency to heal itself is another element of the chiropractic paradigm, its belief in 'naturalness'. Because the body is built to nature's order, and because it has the natural ability to fight off disease, it should not be tampered with by using drugs. Palmer's paradigm was therefore a drugless one. While drugs may affect the symptoms, they will not remedy the cause. The care provider must also look to nature for the cure, and for chiropractors that meant, where possible, no drugs, surgery or other modalities beyond the hand.

The sociological paradigm

A sociological paradigm refers to the social organization of a recognizable social group around a paradigm. Clearly, this happened with chiropractic. Professional and political associations have been formed, schools founded, research foundations established and journals and indexes published, and chiropractors are recognized by statutes in most of the jurisdictions in Western society where they practice. While there are schisms within the profession, some along philosophical lines, and therefore one paradigm cannot strictly be said to dominate the profession, there is enough uniformity for outsiders to recognize the providers as 'chiropractors', and as thereby subscribing to a paradigm more similar to other chiropractors than to non-chiropractors.

The research paradigm

As Kuhn noted, the most productive period for a paradigm in science is the period of normal science, where the major activity is solving puzzles within the terms of reference of the paradigm. There are two important elements here. The first is that the puzzles are those presented by the paradigm itself. For example, puzzles about relativity are important research issues within Einstein's paradigm, but not within Newton's. In the latter it would make no sense to engage in such puzzles, since the paradigm does not incorporate the notion of relativity. This does not mean that those interested in relativity cannot revisit Newton to ponder how the concepts might be reconciled, but it does mean that, prior to Einstein, Newtonian physics was not engaged in solving problems about relativity. So in a real sense, the paradigm and its associated puzzles lay out a research programme for scientists to follow. These puzzles may be thought of as the 'what if' questions' of the paradigm – for example, what if

Einstein is right about relativity? What predictions might that lead us to? What experiments should we conduct to test them out? What answers would be acceptable?

The second element is that scientists, during normal periods of science, attempt to apply the paradigm across as wide a spectrum of puzzles as possible, to solve all that they can with the paradigm. As long as scientists continue to do so successfully, any counter-evidence that might challenge the very validity of the paradigm is ignored and, for Kuhn, should be ignored.

Following this logic of paradigm development in science, the natural consequence of Palmer's paradigm should have been the development of a research programme. Until very recently, chiropractic did not produce a period of normal science [7]. Since there was nothing inherent in the paradigm of D. D. Palmer that would have mitigated the development of a research paradigm, its failure to do so provides an interesting puzzle.

The reasons it did not are complex, and form part of the history of chiropractic. To establish itself, chiropractic was forced very quickly to develop an identity that would distinguish it from other practices such as osteopathy. To do this, it rapidly became focused on the metaphysical and philosophical elements of the paradigm, which soon became dogmatic and ideological. Chiropractic was also very soon under attack from medicine, with chiropractors being prosecuted for practising medicine without a licence. A major defence was to claim that chiropractic was a distinct branch of the healing arts. Since the ailments they treated were not distinct, and neither was the therapy, the major distinction became the 'intent' for which they gave the adjustment. Lacking a scientific rationale for this so early in the development of the paradigm, chiropractors turned to so-called chiropractic philosophy, metaphysics and dogma for their legal defence [8]. Had chiropractic not encountered such adamant political and legal opposition virtually from the moment of its creation, and had it not been successful in using the 'philosophical defence', it is likely the outcome might have been different and a genuine research paradigm might have had the opportunity to emerge during the early history of chiropractic.

Chiropractic isolation from mainstream educational institutions also hurt chiropractic in this regard. As health itself moved increasingly towards health science within the university setting, and as the full intellectual and economic resources were applied to the development of these sciences, chiropractic, as did all the alternative health professions, fell further and further behind in the area of research. In many ways this became a vicious cycle. Without inclusion in research institutions, chiropractic was left either to fund and conduct all its own research (a feat certainly not accomplished by medicine) or to withdraw from it altogether. Of course, without any credible research and scholarship chiropractors were then denied membership in the very institutions that might have allowed them to overcome this lack. For most of its history, the chiropractic profession decided to disengage from research and, although this has changed, it is only in the last 30 years that any appreciable paradigm research has occurred. The profession also developed a very strong anti-intellectual bias from a very early period, under the leadership of B. J. Palmer.

Conclusions

In conclusion, then, the lack of a research paradigm historically is more correctly an issue of abstinence than impotence. This does not mean that chiropractic has not been informed by research throughout its history. Chiropractic education has always included an extensive programme in the basic biological sciences, and chiropractic writings have drawn on the scientific literature. However, for the most part, chiropractic has had to turn to other disciplines and other research paradigms to provide scientific rationales for its own paradigm. This is reflected in the fact that the textbooks used in chiropractic education, particularly during the first two years, are overwhelmingly written by non-chiropractors. It is also reflected in the fact that, until very recently, chiropractic lacked indexed, peer-reviewed scientific journals, research foundations and literature databases. However, a major transformation has occurred in the last 30 years, and this is described below.

The contemporary research paradigm

While chiropractic has been politically marginalized by medicine throughout much of its history, it has been able to establish itself in the current health-care system mainly through political means and patient loyalty. A lack of scientific evidence, while it has hindered acceptance, has not prevented what may now be termed the mainstreaming of chiropractic[9]. It may, however, explain the slowness with which the research paradigm has developed. The experience of the chiropractic profession suggests that knowledge, and different types of knowledge, play varying roles at different historical periods in legitimating social groups. It also suggests that the social/cultural context will determine in a large part what that role will be. Until very recently, it could be said that chiropractic was legitimated not because of research, but in spite of it. As seen below, this may no longer be true.

For much of its history, the information available about chiropractic was either written by chiropractors proselytizing the practice or by medical doctors denigrating it. From the 1950s onwards, a new group, social scientists, began researching chiropractors. There is an extensive list of publications spanning these 40 years in sociology and anthropology. The early sociological writings on chiropractic were characterized by an interest in the esoteric features of the profession[10]. The focus was on the assumed marginality of chiropractic, its cultism, its professionalism or lack of it, and its deviant theory of disease. This earlier body of literature in the social sciences gives very little factual information about chiropractic. The social sciences were initially less concerned with a systematic empirical account of chiropractic and more concerned with the conceptualization of the role or the profession in society, and theorizing either about the causes or the effects of that role.

From the 1970s[11] onwards, a change occurred in the social science writings on chiropractic. Writers were increasingly likely to acknowledge that the earlier conceptualizations of chiropractic as marginal were not based on empirical data, and to acknowledge that the focus on marginality was no longer appropriate – that it was, in all likelihood, a politically created marginality. They were also more likely to entertain the idea of chiropractic as a distinct paradigm. More recently, a body of work in the social sciences has examined chiropractic in relation to medical dominance, and recognizes the political nature of much of the opposition. An increasing number of social scientists publish in chiropractic journals[12].

A rapidly growing body of literature on chiropractic services is also developing in the area of health services research. One major area of interest here has been the comparison of medical and chiropractic care. The health services literature is also using empirical data to test various hypotheses about chiropractic utilization and its role in health care. Other areas include the efficacy of chiropractic (and spinal manipulation) in clinical trials (meta-analyses), and the appropriateness of spinal manipulation and the economics of chiropractic care[13]. Increasingly this research is being conducted by the chiropractic profession itself, in conjunction with them, or funded by them. It is also increasingly being published in non-chiropractic scholarly journals.

Recent and current research

Chiropractic is unique amongst the alternative health professions in the degree to which it has instituted research in recent years. In the United States there now exist two major research foundations funded by the profession – the Foundation for Chiropractic Education and Research, and the Consortium for Chiropractic Research – and several minor ones. In addition, all accredited chiropractic colleges are mandated by the Council on Chiropractic Education (the accrediting agency) to have a division of research. The profession has several international research journals and, in the United States, the *Journal of Manipulative and Physiological Therapeutics* is indexed in *Index Medicus*. There now exist library databases, the Chiropractic Literature Analysis and Retrieval System (CHIROLARS), and the Index to Chiropractic Literature (ICL), for accessing chiropractic literature and research. Last but not least, in the United States the US Department of Health and Human Services, Health Resources and Services Administration (HRSA) has conducted three major national workshops (and are planning a fourth) with the objective of developing a chiropractic research agenda. The National Institutes for Health, through the Office of Alternative Medicine, is currently funding a Consortial Center for Chiropractic Research.

Along with this new emphasis on the research paradigm has come increased scrutiny of chiropractic by researchers. At the very point at which chiropractic history becomes engaged in research, medicine and mainstream health care is entering an era of evidence-based practice. While it has taken all of this century for medicine to reach this point, chiropractic is being catapulted into it in the very early stages of its research development. Three recently published studies illustrate in a dramatic way how this change impacts on the chiropractic profession. The first study appeared in the *Annals of Internal Medicine*[14]. This study estimated the rate of appropriateness of the use of manipulation for low back pain in chiropractic clinics. While the study showed that manipulation was used inappropriately on 29 per cent of the patients, it also noted that this was comparable to rates of inappropriate care for carotid endarterectomy (32 per cent) and coronary artery bypass graft surgery (14 per cent). Some of the press tended to highlight the fact that 29 per cent of manipulations were inappropriate, and not that 46 per cent were judged to be appropriate. The study was widely quoted in the press, but in a variety of ways. A number were positive reports: *Chiropractic gains support. Study shows growing acceptance of alternative treatments for back pain; Chiropractic is good care, a study says; Study gives nod to chiropractic benefits; Getting the kinks out. Chiropractors are effective in nearly half of bad-back cases, researchers say; Study: Chiropractic works in nearly half of back cases;* and *Study gives chiropractors a vote of confidence.* However, other reports were presented negatively: *Study revives debate on manipulation for low back pain relief; Study: 1 in 4 chiropractic treatments inappropriate;* and *Spinal manipulation study draws criticism.*

The *New England Journal of Medicine*, in October 1998, published two articles critical of chiropractic care. The first was a study of the contribution of chiropractic to the treatment of asthma[15], showing in effect that the addition of chiropractic care to children with mild or moderate asthma provided no benefit. The second study[16] reported on a trial comparing chiropractic with the McKenzie method of physical therapy and the provision of an educational booklet. The patients getting either chiropractic or physical therapy had only marginally better outcomes than those getting the booklet, but incurred much greater costs (the physical therapy cost was slightly higher than chiropractic). Once again this study was widely quoted in the media, but with a different slant – *Chiropractic's success on back pain disputed in study;* and *Challenging the main reason people go to chiropractors, a major medical journal today is releasing a study showing that spinal manipulation eases back pain no better than physical therapy and only a bit better than doing next to nothing.* In none of the headlines was physical therapy actually mentioned, even though the study was as concerned with this as much as chiropractic.

Up until this point in time, the reviews of the trials done on manipulation[17] had largely supported the efficacy of this form of therapy or had been inconclusive. This most recent work in the area of health services research poses a quite different social challenge to chiropractic. For the most part, the work in anthropology was published in non-health journals, was unlikely to be quoted in the press, and was even less likely to be read by the chiropractic patient. For the most part, this literature was not available to chiropractors. Within the educational community, the community of scholars, these articles clearly influenced how chiropractic was viewed, and they were quoted when government bodies were examining chiropractic legislatively.

However, health services research has a totally different audience. It is widely read by those involved in delivering health care and those funding it. The results are increasingly available to the community, and the media picks it up and will place 'interest' pieces on the front page (often distorting the results in the process). Therefore, as the inclusion of chiropractic in health services research increases, so does the political cost. On the one hand, such research has clearly contributed to the mainstreaming of chiropractic; on the other, it also threatens it. What are the likely responses? Some preliminary comments can be made. A major response has been to challenge the narrow focus and, in some cases, the research designs. A broader response, however, has been to challenge the research paradigms being used. This is a philosophical issue that has its counterpart in the interpretative social sciences and in such areas as nursing, where the fundamental critique is the appropriateness of a reductionist, positivist-empiricist paradigm for researching a holistic health encounter.

Conclusion

The conclusion drawn from chiropractic history is that the relationship of knowledge to the social legitimation of a health paradigm is a complex and changing process, and is also heavily influenced by the social historical context. In earlier periods, chiropractic was able successfully to counter challenges to the legitimacy of its paradigm caused by lack of research. The writings in sociology and anthropology that could have harmed the legitimacy were not written by groups who were socially powerful. While medicine provided a powerful group, and its labelling of chiropractic as quackery obviously affected the legitimacy of chiropractic, the work was clearly prejudiced and self-serving and, because chiropractic patients tended to be persons fleeing from medicine for particular conditions, chiropractors were able successfully to overcome the opposition through political action and patient loyalty.

However, with the development of their own research paradigm and their involvement in health services research, chiropractors face an entirely new challenge. First, this type of research is largely carried out without prejudice to any single group within the health field. Stated another way, health services research is not doing anything to chiropractic that it has not already done or is doing to medicine. Second, in an historical age where health-care costs tend to drive the system, and where the dominant ideology is that only those things that can be shown to be efficacious or cost-effective should be funded, the chiropractic profession needs this research to justify itself. As noted earlier, much of the work is being conducted by individuals in the profession and, even when this is not the case, is being funded by the profession. In an era where evidence-based practice is the mantra, the complementary and alternative health-care providers are vulnerable to a new form of evaluation. Where once patient satisfaction might have sufficed, measurable outcomes are now required. While for much of their history chiropractors have successfully operated outside mainstream health care, a new economic order confronts them. Alternative and complementary health care is increasingly covered by health insurance. As with the mainstream health professionals, alternative providers are increasingly experiencing the insertion of third party payers between them and their patients.

The paradigm concept therefore provides a way in which to think about chiropractic and to pose interesting questions such as the failure, until recently, to give rise to a productive research tradition. It also provides a concept for examining chiropractic *vis-à-vis* other health paradigms, highlighting some of the similarities and continuities but also isolating the differences. Looked at from the perspective of a paradigm, chiropractic seems no more irrational, dogmatic or ideological than other paradigms that have populated science and health; nor does it seem any less so. While it appears that it has developed a research programme somewhat late, it has only just celebrated its 100-year anniversary. One could argue that medicine, around since ancient Greece, has taken considerably longer to develop its own impressive research paradigm(s), and has incorporated the notion of evidence-based practice only in the last part of the twentieth century. Seen in that time frame, one might argue that the chiropractic paradigm has emerged as a research paradigm with considerable speed.

References

[1] Kuhn, T. (1962). *The Structure of Scientific Revolutions*. University Chicago Press.

[2] Coulter, I. D. (1992). *The defense of Thomas Kuhn (and chiropractic). J. Manipul. Physiol. Ther.*, **15(6)**, 392–401.

[3] Kuhn, T (1974). Second thought on paradigms. In *The Structure of Scientific Theories* (P. Suppe, ed.), pp. 459–82. University of Illinois Press.

[4] Masterman, M. (1970). The nature of a paradigm. In *Criticism and the Growth of Knowledge* (I. Lakatos and A. Musgrave, eds), pp. 58–89. Cambridge University Press.

[5] Donahue, J. D. (1987). D. D. Palmer and the metaphysical movement in the nineteenth century. *Chiropr. Hist.*, **7**, 23–7.

[6] Coulter, I. D. (1990). The chiropractic paradigm. *J. Manipul. Physiol. Ther.*, **13(5)**, 279–87.

[7] Coulter, I. D. (1991). Philosophy of science and chiropractic research. *J. Manipul. Physiol. Ther.*, **14(4)**, 269–71.

[8] Richards, D. M. (1991). The Palmer philosophy of chiropractic – an historical perspective. *Chiropr. J. Aust.*, **21(2)**, 63–7.

[9] Coulter, I. D. (1996). The role of the chiropractor in the changing health-care system: from marginal to mainstream. *Res. Sociol. Health Care*, **13A**, 95–117.

[10] Coulter, I. D. (1991). Sociological studies of the role of the chiropractor: an exercise in ideological hegemony. *J. Manipul. Physiol. Ther.*, **14(1)**, 51–8.

[11] Coulter, I. D. (1983). Chiropractic observed: thirty years of a changing sociological perspective. *Chiropr. Hist.*, **3**, 43–7.

[12] Coulter, I. D. (1992). The sociology of chiropractic: future options and directions. In *Principles and Practice of Chiropractic* (S. Haldeman, ed.), pp. 53–9. Appleton and Lange.

[13] Mootz, R. D., Coulter, I. D. and Hansen D. T. (1997). Health services research related to chiropractic: review and recommendations for research prioritization by the chiropractic profession. *J. Manipul. Physiol. Ther.*, **20(3)**, 201–21.

[14] Shekelle, P. G., Coulter, I. D., Hurwitz, E. L. *et al.* (1998). Congruence between decisions to initiate chiropractic spinal manipulation for low back pain and appropriateness criteria in North America. *Ann. Int. Med.*, **129(1)**, 9–17.

[15] Balon, J., Aker, P. D., Crowther, E. R. *et al.* (1998). A comparison of active and simulated chiropractic manipulation as adjunctive treatment for childhood asthma. *New Engl. J. Med.*, **339(5)**, 1013–19.

[16] Cherkin, D.C., Deyo R. A., Battie M. *et al.* (1998). A comparison of physical therapy, chiropractic manipulation, and provision of an educational booklet for the treatment of patients with low back pain. *New Engl. J. Med.*, **339(15)**, 1021–9.

[17] Coulter, I. D. (1998). Efficacy and risks of chiropractic manipulation: what does the evidence suggest? *Integr. Med.*, **1(2)**, 61–6.

Metaphysical matters

Metaphysics in chiropractic and alternative health care

As we have seen in the previous chapters, the chiropractic paradigm has been characterized by the strong role that metaphysical beliefs have played in its development. However, as noted, conflict over metaphysical matters has given rise to two contending visions of chiropractic, termed the innatists and the rationalists. Where the former embrace the metaphysic of vitalism, the latter eschew any role for metaphysics. In fact, both camps misconstrue the nature and role of metaphysics; the innatists by assuming that metaphysical beliefs cannot be subjected to philosophical critique and change, and that they are inviolate, and the rationalists by assuming that metaphysics cannot be part of science[1]. The history of science demonstrates the absurdity of the latter belief. Yesterday's metaphysic, such as the belief that the sun is the centre of the universe, initially a belief for the cult of sun worshippers, is today's science (the heliocentric universe). At the same time, the belief that the earth was the centre of the universe (a geocentric universe), which was considered science up until the time of Copernicus, can become tomorrow's metaphysical belief. Science itself constitutes a metaphysical belief system based on *a priori* assumptions not amenable to proof. These include a belief in causation (an intellectual construction that is inferred from observing events), a belief that we can discover causes, a belief that only the five senses are legitimate for collecting data from which to infer causation, a belief that reason and logic are the most powerful intellectual methods for organizing such data, and a belief that replication and consensus are the best methods for establishing a scientific fact.

Not only has this conflict over metaphysical beliefs caused considerable difficulty within the profession; it has also frequently hurt the profession externally. Probably more than any other single element of the paradigm, the metaphysical elements have often given chiropractic the appearance of a religious dogma. In this regard, chiropractic suffers from the same problem as many, if not all, the alternative health paradigms, most of which subscribe to some form of vitalism. Historically, such beliefs have been counterpoised with those of science in medicine. A critical confrontation with this issue is therefore important, not only in understanding chiropractic but also in understanding alternative health care generally.

Vitalism

Within philosophy, vitalism is generally portrayed as a failed metaphysic. Kekes[2], for example, has argued that the demise of vitalism was due to death by a thousand qualifications. He felt that vitalism had been seriously weakened, although not proven false, by biological materialism. If all illness and disease can be explained empirically by biological determinism, metaphysical systems that input such concepts as vitalistic forces become irrelevant. If 'life' can be explained in material terms in the same way that non-living phenomena can, then the major distinction of vitalism loses its force. If no difference exists between inanimate and animate objects in terms of scientific analysis, the very philosophical justification for vitalism becomes suspect. It is not so much a question of vitalism not being true, as a question of it not being needed. For Kekes, this also implied that the ontological presuppositions of vitalism need to be abandoned.

Science and metaphysics

Metaphysics, in introducing the conceptual model as an articulate, explicit object of criticism, represents the way back to a critique of the foundations of our understanding ... When a metaphysic holds itself immune from a critique then it degenerates into non-metaphysical ritual and dogma.

Wartofsky[3]

Metaphysics are part of science, and play the dominant role in determining which scientific problems within a period will be engaged by the scientists[4] (in Kuhn's terms, they determine the puzzles of normal science). Under this view, metaphysics can be seen as the basis of research programmes, setting the research agenda. Metaphysics are heuristics for both theory and research, and form the basis for articulating alternative conceptual schemes.

However, because they are articulated systematized schema, they can also be criticized. Since metaphysics can be formalized, they must have some relationship to logic. Metaphysics all claim to be an interpretation of the world, all claim to be rational, and most claim to be true, even if they are unsure how this could be determined. Also, since there can be alternative metaphysics that contradict them, they must possibly be false. The hope for a genuine science lies not in jettisoning the metaphysical past, but in critical confrontation with it[3].

Metaphysics in science

Before discussing the issue of how to critique metaphysics in science, it is useful to consider what constitutes a metaphysic, the important role they have played in science and their fall from grace[1]. Metaphysics are broad generalizations about the nature of the world, and are usually ontological (about the ultimate nature of reality). Unlike theories that try to make sense of observations, metaphysics are *a priori* in that they provide schemes in terms of which reality can be approached before we even begin to think about theory. They are attempts to understand reality at the most general level and, in many ways, they act like metaphors in our language[5]. The purpose of a metaphor is not to state a fact about something, but to provide an alternative way of viewing something within which we might begin to state facts. Both metaphysics and metaphors formulate conditions under which it is possible to state facts. For example, the metaphysic of mechanism in science has the *a priori* postulate that the world is a machine (a metaphor). Under this postulate, Newton was able to develop powerful theories about the nature of that machine and its functioning The metaphor/metaphysic frames the theories and the research programme of Newtonian physics. Similarly, Descartes dualism has the *a priori* assumption that the body is like a machine but the mind is not, and therefore there are two distinct levels of reality. So metaphysics then are statements about reality; not a different reality, but a reality differently conceived[6]. In a sense, just as we do with metaphors, we pretend one thing is something else. So we say, in effect, 'let us pretend that the world is a machine, or that the brain is a computer, or that the world is indeterminate', etc. Then, if that is the case, we ask what predictions we can make; 'what if the world is a machine?'. The 'what if' questions may simply be logically derived as they are in Euclid geometry. For example, if two parallel lines do not meet, what can we predict about a right-angled triangle? Other examples of metaphysics in science besides mechanism and dualism include realism, idealism, materialism, reductionism, instrumentalism, uniformitarianism, functionalism, structuralism, determinism and indeterminacy. These are all fundamental presuppositions whose truth or falsehood cannot be established empirically through observation. They are also fundamental in the sense that the purpose of research done under their guidance is not to question or test these assumptions. To this extent, they are the taken-for-granted guidelines for investigation. If they are challenged, it will be through an appeal to alternative metaphysics. So, for example, Descartes challenges the extreme notion of mechanism, and rescues mechanism, by establishing a dualism to deal with the order of the mind. Current chaos theory challenges the metaphysic of determinacy.

Despite the obvious importance of metaphysics in science, they have not been accorded a very important role by either contemporary scientists or the philosophy of science. In classical philosophy, metaphysics was considered the fundamental and most general science, the science of first principles. In many ways, the continuing presence of metaphysics has been something of an embarrassment within science. Historians, philosophers and scientists have no difficulty in recognizing the metaphysics of previous ages, but have tended to argue that mature science involves their eradication, and portray early instances as ignorance on the part of scientists. If metaphysics is given any role, it is in the area of scientific discovery but not in scientific justification. The attempt to portray metaphysics as an historical phenomenon, what yesterday's scientists were influenced by, or to maintain that mature science is characterized by the eradication of metaphysics, has proven to be singularly unsuccessful, as even the most cursory examination of contemporary physics or astronomy would show. In these two sciences, at least, it could be argued that they are becoming more metaphysical rather than less so.

Part of the problem in the philosophy of science was that the logical/empiricist school saw as their central purpose the elimination of metaphysics, which they perceived as empirically meaningless and hence non-scientific, or even anti-scientific. Descarte's dualism also placed all non-physical questions outside the domain of natural philosophy (science) on metaphysical grounds (the mind/body split), which also had the effect of eliminating metaphysical questions from science. However, major metaphysical questions still haunt science. The debate between realism – that is, that science is about reality and truth, and reality is independent of our perception of it – and instrumentalism – that is, science is about our experience and is simply an instrument to order that experience – still rages. These metaphysics have been termed haunted universe doctrines[7]. They are neither analytic nor empirical statements. While they are disguised statements about the world, they really function as guidelines or methodological prescriptions that direct the scientist to look for certain things. Metaphysics is therefore the branch of philosophy that makes explicit, and critiques *a priori* assumptions.

Use of metaphysics in science

The best way to think of metaphysics is to see them as heuristics in science[3]; as devices that are either useful or not useful, rather than true or not true. Clearly they are not static, carved in stone. Yesterday's metaphysic can become today's science. Furthermore, there are some rules/conventions about their use in science.

Metaphysics are eligible for critique and debate. As part of rational discourse, they should at least be rationally controlled visions of the world and, while not empirically confirmable, should give rise to theories and hypotheses that can be empirically examined. Although no single empirical test can, strictly speaking, disprove a metaphysical belief, an accumulation of disproved hypotheses should lead to a critical evaluation of the metaphysical assumptions. Kekes[2] has argued that, as part of rational discourse, they must be logically consistent, have conceptual coherence, have some explanatory power and lead to the solving of some puzzles within the domain in which they occur (in this case, health). In science, they are judged by the extent to which they give rise to a successful programme of research. So, for example, while the metaphysical systems underlying most of biomedicine (mechanism, reductionism and biological determinism) may be criticized on numerous grounds, and are now being challenged as the appropriate philosophical grounding for medicine, they did give rise to a highly successful research paradigm. That is, they did contribute significantly to solving health puzzles. Furthermore, although not confirmable, the metaphysics should be capable of specifying conditions which, if held true, would count as a falsification, a disproof. The latter condition may not be possible to achieve until some time in the future. This is the situation that has occurred with sub-atomic particles, where much of the disproving has had to wait on the development of techniques to investigate this order of reality. Since the metaphysics in science are intended as statements about reality, and usually intended as true statements, they must also be capable of describing a reality incompatible with the one they describe.

In science, therefore, metaphysics are heuristic devices that, while we may not be able to say they are true or false, can be judged useful or non-useful. The extent to which they are useful is the extent to which they expand our knowledge, and the extent to which they solve puzzles. However, Kekes[2] believes that initially no meta-physical theory could survive such a rigorous evaluation and, therefore, that they should not be given up too readily. It makes sense to stick with the metaphysic, even in the face of initial shortcomings. Even if the metaphysic survives a critical evaluation, we still do not know if it is true; we know that it has survived a critique. Furthermore, contradictory or mutually exclusive metaphysics may co-exist. The point is, they can be rationally debated. It is when they do not become part of a critical tradition, when they hold themselves immune to critique, that they have the greatest potential to do harm. When the *a priori* assumptions of metaphysical system are isolated and made explicit, they can become objects for intellectual scrutiny and rational debate. The problem with them is that they can readily degenerate into pseudo-science or mysticism. What was perhaps a brilliant insight degenerates into dogma, what was debatable becomes doctrine, and what was an heuristic device becomes a hegemonic one[1]. To understand this we need to understand the role of metaphors in science, because it is in the form of metaphors that metaphysics are expressed and incorporated into scientific thinking. In essence, metaphysics provide the root metaphors for scientific paradigms.

Metaphors and science

The relationship between metaphors and metaphysics is such that metaphysical beliefs are expressed in terms of metaphors ('the world is a machine' is the metaphorical expression of the metaphysic mechanism), and each metaphor in science has, as its root, a fundamental metaphysic. Furthermore, it is in the form of metaphors that metaphysics run the danger of becoming myths. This occurs when the metaphor, in a sense, goes underground, and persons using the metaphor lose sight of the fact that it is a metaphor. What begins as a possible truth (the world is like a machine) comes to be seen as the literal truth (the world is a machine) and, even worse, the only possible truth. This is a process of reification, whereby an heuristic device created by scientists for investigating the world comes to be seen as other than this, and begins to convert to determining how persons see the world – that is, it is viewed as an empirical scientific truth about the world. The metaphors come to have a life of their own. It is one thing to describe the world as *like* a machine, but another to believe it *is* a machine. The difference between a metaphor and a myth is that with the former we make-believe something is true, while in the latter we believe it. To the extent that we see it as the only truth, we blind ourselves to seeing other possibilities.

The danger occurs because, as the metaphor goes underground, we lose sight of the implicit assumptions that accompany the metaphor, and they now become fixed assumptions that are often unrecognized, undefined and uncriticized. This can be seen very readily in language, where we lose sight of the fact that to describe something as, for example, the 'foot of the mountain' is, in fact, to use a metaphor. However, on challenging the speaker ('how do you mean, the foot of the mountain?') we immediately become conscious not only of the fact that it is a metaphor, but also that its meaning can be contested. Clearly, the bottom of a mountain is not at all like a foot. With metaphors, we can choose to use them as heuristic devices, and also run the risk of being used by them – that is, we become victims of our own metaphors. While metaphors can often be acceptable absurdities (clearly the bottom of a mountain is not a foot), myths are dangerous because they become believed absurdities. To understand this, we need to understand a little about metaphors themselves.

The importance of metaphors

There is a long history of discussions about metaphors in philosophy, going as far back as Aristotle[5]. A metaphor involves seeing, describing or portraying one thing as something else. In language, it involves calling one thing by the name of another. Theories about metaphors have examined the relationship between the two terms; the subject and the modifier. This relationship has been described as a contradiction, a logical absurdity, a factual absurdity, a metaphorical twist, sort crossing, and a category mistake. It involves calling something by another name when it is obvious, both to the speaker and the listener, that it is not the thing named. It is an apparent absurdity that we choose to accept as being intended by the speaker (a deliberate category mistake), and therefore it must have another meaning that we must search for (although in a good metaphor we tend to jump directly to the new meaning; it seems self-evident). Metaphors have the tremendous advantage of allowing us to say something new, but to say it within our present language[6]. They are clearly an integral part of the process by which we expand our meanings, and also our understanding. In one sense, all new knowledge (in science or elsewhere) is metaphorical. We can only know the unknown in terms of the known, which means we can only get new knowledge through metaphorical extension of our language[8]. We express our understanding through the language we have. Even if we come up with a totally new word (e.g. 'quarks'), it must still be defined in terms of our existing language. However, our language imposes restrictions on its literal use. Simply put, if we wish to say some things literally in our language, we cannot say other things without inconsistency (e.g. 'I'd like half a dozen, but not six'). Metaphors, on the other hand, allow us to use the same words for inconsistent use. To call a person a pig is not possible if we wish to remain literal, but is entirely possible if we are being metaphorical.

Unfortunately, despite the importance of metaphors they have been treated in much the same way in science and philosophy as metaphysics generally, and relegated to the discovery process only. Bunge[9] reflects this attitude in the following: 'To suggest that scientific explanation is metaphorical is to mistake scientific theories for biblical parables or to subscribe to instrumentalism'. Mature science involves replacing metaphors with literal statements in this view. Metaphors pose a unique challenge to philosophers of science since they seem to suggest that scientific knowledge, truth, arises out of contradictions or absurdities. To accept a metaphorical theory of science would be to accept that scientific truth arises out of initial falsehood a position which challenges directly some of the major functions of a philosophy of science, the clarification of thought, the resolving of contradictions, and the eradication of absurdities and category mistakes. Metaphors have largely been seen in the philosophy of science as subjective, emotive elements.

Critical appraisal of metaphors in science

If metaphors and metaphysics are an inherent part of science, the challenge for both scientists and philosophers is, what criteria can we establish for their rational criticism? In some ways, the field of aesthetics already does this. In literary criticism it is quite clear that we are able to distinguish the creative, fresh metaphors of Shakespeare from, say, a trite metaphor. The challenge is explaining the meaning of the metaphor. One principle[10] is the principle of congruence; what are the permissible connotations of the metaphor? A second principle is plentitude, whereby all connotations that could fit the particular context are attributed (it means all it can mean). Within literature, we tend to be critical of mixed metaphors. Good metaphors are more complex than banal or trite metaphors. They seem to say more about a topic, and in an original and insightful way, they are more discriminating and precise.

In many ways, however, the problem is no different to that of judging a hypothesis in science. In one sense, a metaphor is a hypothesis. For example to say 'love is a red, red rose' is to hypothesize about love. In science, a hypothesis is judged by its ability to account for the greatest quantity of phenomena – does it explain as much as possible? We also use the principle of parsimony or simplicity, and choose the hypothesis that explains the most with the least variables. Good hypotheses tend to be bold conjectures[11], which imply more consequences and are therefore more readily falsified. They also lead to a proliferation of sub-hypotheses. Metaphors can be judged, as can hypotheses, in terms of saving the most appearances: which ones account for the generally agreed facts, or which ones account for the most facts? Which metaphors lead to the development of new tests? Which ones best account for the existing puzzles?

Metaphors and myths

The greatest challenge, however, is in distinguishing metaphor from myths. This requires three analytical steps. The first involves showing that the scientist is no longer conscious that it is a metaphor. The second step involves demonstrating that the metaphor has gone 'underground'. This can be shown to occur when assumptions are transposed by the metaphor from the old to the new, these can be isolated in the new theory, their presence is unexplained or undefined, and they are clearly predicated on the metaphor itself[9]. In this case, the process of reification has clearly occurred. Last but not least, the third step involves assessing whether the implicit assumptions are distortions – whether the metaphor suppresses or leaves out readily available evidence about the phenomenon in question.

The source of metaphors can also be the basis for criticism. This is clearly seen in the social sciences, where to use mechanistic metaphors to describe humans can be seen as dehumanizing. At various times, different sources have provided the metaphors so that a physical heart can become the heart of the matter, and the political state can become the state of equilibrium of the body. Technology has provided very powerful metaphors (a pump, computer, telephone exchange) for describing the body. Since you cannot conceive of the heart as a pump until a pump has been invented, it was once seen as a furnace. War becomes the war on cancer. Even within basic science, however, the source of metaphors can become problematic. The pursuit of physical determinism in mechanical terms, when it is clear that atoms sometimes behave like particles but at other times can best be described in terms of wave equations, becomes a barrier to our understanding.

Two other problems come from the use of animation (e.g. 'the jaws of hell') and anthropomorphism (giving non-human objects human qualities) in metaphors. While in literature these can be effective, in science they pose the same problem as generalizing from animal studies to humans. The danger is that a normative statement comes to be mistaken for a descriptive one.

Conclusion

In this chapter we have attempted to use philosophy to clarify the role of metaphysics and metaphors. The purpose was to establish that metaphysics have a role in science, but that they must form part of a critical debate. Where this does not occur, myth and dogma results. In chiropractic, as in all the alternative health paradigms, the real test of the metaphysics of both the innatist and rationalist positions is a pragmatic one. Does invoking the concepts of universal and innate intelligence give rise to a productive investigative paradigm, does it lead to significant expansion of our knowledge, and does it solve health puzzles with more explanatory power than competing concepts? The same questions can be asked of the rationalists. Concepts such as innate and universal intelligence are metaphors. In some ways they are animated metaphors, ascribing intelligence to physiological processes. However, as metaphors they are simply an expression of a much more fundamental metaphysical belief, that of vitalism.

The essential feature of vitalism is that it posits a distinction between living and non-living things. In positivistic philosophy, writers such as Francis Bacon rejected forces that were not observable. Descartes also insisted that the body obeyed the same physical laws as the rest of the universe. Newtonian physics argued that all matter obeyed physical laws, and that these were predictable. When applied to biology, as explanations more and more frequently evoked physiochemical factors to describe the functioning of the body, the need for vitalism disappeared. However, vitalism itself did not disappear, and was kept alive in the alternative health paradigms. Partly because of their belief in holism, these paradigms have always argued against the reductionism involved in the biomedical paradigm, asserting instead that the whole is more than the sum of its parts. They also embraced the idea that the body functions to heal itself, and that its natural state is one of health. It does this through mechanisms of homeostasis. Until the recent advent of psychoneuro-immunology, the only way to account for this natural healing tendency was to invoke the notion of vitalism (innate). The alternative paradigms were left very much like chiropractic; the philosophy of chiropractic of health and healing required a concept such as vitalism to make it work. Chiropractors, however, lacked both the training in philosophy to establish an acceptable intellectual formulation of the concept, and a research paradigm that might have been able to establish it as a useful heuristic. Such a paradigm would have given rise to a productive research programme (a period of puzzle-solving normal science). Vitalism therefore became what we identified earlier as a major danger, the dogma and myth of chiropractic.

References

[1] Coulter, I. D. (1993). Metaphysics, rationality and science. *J. Manipul. Physiol. Ther.*, **16(5)**, 319–26.
[2] Kekes, J. (1973). The rationality of metaphysics. *Metaphilosophy*, **4**, 124–39.
[3] Wartofsky, N. W. (1967). Metaphysics as an heuristic for science. In *Boston Studies in the Philosophy of Science III* (R. S. Cohen and M. W. Wartofsky, eds), pp. 123–72. Reidel Publishing Company.
[4] Agassi, J. (1964). The nature of scientific problems and their roots in metaphysics. In *The Critical Approach to Science and Philosophy* (M. Bunge, ed.), pp. 189–211. Free Press.
[5] Coulter, I. D. (1990). Of clouds and clocks and chiropractors: toward a theory of irrationality. *Am. J. Chiro. Med.*, **3(2)**, 84–92.
[6] Stewart, D. B. (1972). *The Concept of Metaphor*. PhD thesis, University of London.
[7] Watkins, J. W. N. (1958). Confirmable and influential metaphysics. *Mind*, **LXVII**, 344–65.
[8] Schon, D. A. (1963). *Development of Concepts*. Tavistock Publications.
[9] Bunge, M. (1968). Analogy in quantum theory. From insight to nonsense. *Br. J. Philos.* **18**, 265–86.
[10] Beardsley, M. C. (1962). The metaphorical twist. *Philos. Phenomenol. Res.*, **XXII**, 293–307.
[11] Popper, K. R. (1969) *Conjectures and Refutations. The Growth of Scientific Knowledge*. Routledge and Kegan Paul.

CHAPTER 4

A philosophy of chiropractic

Throughout the book we have referred to so-called 'chiropractic philosophy' as a misnomer and have argued that, where it is actually philosophical, it should more correctly be termed the philosophy of chiropractic. A strong philosophy of chiropractic would help to answer important questions, such as: What is the nature and purpose of chiropractic? What kinds of concepts populate chiropractic, and how do they explain disease, illness, health, treatment and cure? What kind of science is chiropractic? What is the nature of the clinical art of chiropractic? What kind of values does chiropractic embrace?[1] However, chiropractic was not developed in a vacuum, and it partakes of many intellectual sources. In one sense, chiropractic can be seen historically as drawing from several distinct philosophical sources: vitalism, holism, naturalism, therapeutic conservatism, humanism and critical rationalism[2,3]. By examining each, we can begin to answer the questions posed above.

Vitalism

Part of the difficulty in clarifying the role of vitalism in chiropractic is that chiropractors have used a variety of terms to express this concept. Bryner[4] has noted that 'innate intelligence, as part of broader universal intelligence, is variously used interchangeably with soul, spirit, spark of life, *vis medicatrix naturae*, innate, innate potential, instinct, superconscious, nature, christ-conscious'. This reflects the fact that a metaphysic can have numerous metaphorical expressions, both within chiropractic and across the alternative health-care spectrum.

Vitalism has a very long history in the field of health. It accepts that all living organisms are sustained by a vital force that is both different from and greater than physical and chemical forces. In its extreme form, it assumes that the vital force is supernatural. For many followers of vitalism, the patterns of life and its apparent logic suggest the existence of a higher intelligence. In Palmer's conception, the systems of the body were regulated by an innate intelligence, which was itself an expression of universal intelligence. This metaphysical construct embraces a purposeful, intention-guided, intelligent universe. Since the world seems to obey physical laws and is intelligible, it therefore follows that it must have been created by an intelligent being. Not only is the concept metaphysical, but it is also teleological in that it first posits a world that is purposeful, intention-guided, an intelligent universe, but then uses the existence of such a world as evidence for a universal and innate intelligence. If the world seems to obey physical laws and is therefore intelligible, then it follows it must have been created by an intelligent being. How do we know such a being exists? Because an intelligible world exists.

However, there are expressions of vitalism that do not necessarily imply the presence of a supernatural, intelligent being. An example is captured by the expression *vis medicatrix naturae* (the healing power of nature), which describes the inherent capacity of the body to heal itself, a key postulate in 'chiropractic philosophy'. This form of vitalism is an important part of contemporary chiropractic. Furthermore, it points the way to a unique conception of the practitioner as a facilitator in the healing process, where the true locus of health is the patient. Health comes from within or not at all. It is this philosophical tenet that is shared, implicitly or explicitly, by most chiropractors, and this does not imply a supernatural being. It is important to note therefore that there is both a strong (some would say extreme) and weak form of vitalism.

Within chiropractic, much of the disagreement over the role of vitalism has been premised by the belief that we either accept the radical (supernatural) form of vitalism or reject it all together. Koch[5] has noted that this is a problem of the excluded middle ground of moderate vitalism. This moderate position accepts that nature is an expression of both the physical (material) and the immaterial. The former can and should be empirically studied. However, this material reality is an expression of an organizing principle, and this principle is not captured by the empirical analysis, which captures at best, its expression. As Koch[5] notes, while some chiropractors may personify this in supernatural terms, the concept of vitalism does not demand that we do so. It merely implies that the properties and actions of the material world assume the existence of an organizing principle manifesting itself. While vitalism cannot be empirically investigated, Koch states that 'we can choose to act as if there is a vital, unifying character to life, if we believe this to be the most conducive attitude to adopt in order to fully appreciate life and to interact with other living things most constructively' [5]. Following the critique of metaphysics in the previous chapter, the claim for vitalism needs to be somewhat stronger than this. While Koch himself asks if it has been a hindrance or a help, he is reduced to a very personal criteria for its acceptance. What should be asked is whether vitalism leads to the solution of health problems, the generation of a research programme, or a perception of health and the role of the health provider that makes a difference in the treatment of patients. That is, we are looking for support that would take it beyond a personal theology to a productive philosophy of health care.

Holism

Broadly speaking, holism simply means that the whole is more than the sum of its parts. In health, holism has been defined as 'the balanced integration of the individual in all aspects and levels of being: body, mind and spirit, including interpersonal relationships and our relationships to the whole of nature and our physical environment' [6].

As Gordon notes[7], holism involves recognizing the mental, social, spiritual and physical aspects of the individual, and their importance to health. The notion therefore is that individuals are irreducible units. This, however, implies several things. First, it argues against reductionism. Not only is the whole different to the sum of its parts, but the whole also fundamentally impacts on those parts to the extent that the parts themselves cannot be understood without some reference to the whole. The parts themselves are dynamically interrelated[8]. Korr[9] has isolated three underlying principles that capture holism within a neuromusculoskeletal paradigm such as chiropractic:

1   *The unity of the person*

2   *Vis medicatrix naturae*

3   *Primacy of the musculoskeletal system (or, in chiropractic, the neuromusculoskeletal system).*

In this view, the neuromusculoskeletal system is the means through which we express our uniqueness.

Chiropractic, from its inception, has embraced a holistic philosophy of health. It is based on the concept that the body is an integral unit and that, as long as it maintains this integrity, it is capable of maintaining its own health. The purpose of care is to restore the whole person, not to treat isolated symptoms or diseases. Holism is finding an increasing acceptance within the health sciences as the complex relationship between biology and social/psychological factors comes to be more fully understood, particularly in such fields as pyschoneuroimmunology[10].

Naturalism

D. D. Palmer conceived the body as being built on nature's order. Since the body has by nature the capacity to heal itself, it should not be tampered with unnecessarily through the use of drugs, which may affect the symptoms but do not remove the cause. This implies that we should look to nature for the cure. The body's natural ability to heal is therefore reinforced by the use of natural remedies, and the role of the doctor is to facilitate natural healing. For Palmer, the remedy lay in the therapeutic use of the hands. While an extreme application of this philosophy is virtually untenable in today's society, the preference for natural remedies where appropriate is both philosophically and therapeutically attractive. The so-called wonder drugs have provided near miracles for many of the afflicted, but they (and surgery) have also brought a great increase in iatrogenic illness. Naturalism facilitates a paradigm within health care that is both drugless and non-surgical. There is an increasing public preference for both. For Palmer, the healer 'heals as Nature heals, in accordance with the Nature's laws. Compelling the body to do its own healing with its own forces'[11].

Therapeutic conservatism

The chiropractic paradigm is inherently conservative. This therapeutic approach captures an element expressed by Hippocrates in his directive '*Primum non nocere*' ('First do no harm'). A belief in the body's ability to heal itself (vitalism), in natural therapy (naturalism) and in the whole person (holism) logically implies that the best care is the least care, in the sense that the care provider should use the least amount of intervention necessary to enable the body to heal itself. Under this approach, therapeutic intervention should be directed as much as possible to those things that facilitate the body's own healing capacity. In a world where over-treatment and the use of overly aggressive treatment have become major ethical issues, this philosophical principle has much to recommend it. In addition to the care provider doing as little as possible, this approach is based on the active participation of the patient. So while the provider is exalted to do as little as possible, in one sense the patient is exalted to do as much as possible.

Humanism

Traditionally, humanism is based on the postulate that individuals have immutable rights and, therefore, are worthy of respect for their individuality. An important right, if not the most important, is the right to dignity. In health care, humanism is expressed as concern about the dehumanizing procedures that accompany ill health and in the dehumanizing institutions that have been created to care for the ill. Both impact adversely on the dignity of the patient. Recognition of the personal, social and spiritual aspects of health, and a move away from simply the biology of health, is a manifestation of humanistic principles. A humanistic provider is one who will care for patients, as opposed to one who will simply treat patients – that is, one who is caring. In this perspective, patients are treated with compassion and in settings that reinforce their dignity rather than diminishing it. In chiropractic, this also implies a co-operative relationship with the patient. In a very real sense, it is the patient and the provider together who provide the care for the patient.

Critical rationalism

The philosophy of critical rationalism, largely developed through the work of Karl Popper[12], has been associated with contemporary science and is an important part of the contemporary philosophy of science. It accepts that the universe is amenable to, and can be understood by, reason or rationality; that is, by the methods of scientific investigation used in the natural sciences. The basis of science is the acceptance that reason and logic provide the best intellectual tools for organizing the data collected by the five senses. Science is therefore rational. As propounded by Popper, criticism is the lifeblood of rational thought. Hence, science is critical rationalism.

Critical rationalism as a philosophy embraces several principles[13]. While there is growth in knowledge, all knowledge is provisional. Knowledge improves by elimination of error and by increasing truth, and the ideal of knowledge is that found in science. The essential feature in Popper's notion of science is that hypotheses are falsifiable. In hypotheses, knowledge advances through bold conjectures and refutations by critical assessment. Scientists should be bold in two ways; in their conjectures and in their prediction of consequences, which can be refuted and, if so, lead to falsification of the conjecture. Two other elements are important in this epistemology: all knowledge is fallible (fallibilistic), and all knowledge in principle can be processed further (melioristic).

For Popper, critical rationalism was crucial for the combating of dogma and, therefore, essential for both philosophy and science. All concepts are eligible for comparison and criticism. Those fields with falsifiable concepts are scientific; those that cannot or will not specify the conditions under which their concepts, hypotheses or theories would be refuted are not. Critical rationalism proposes that science should involve the proliferation of bold conjectures, but that all should be subjected to falsification. Without the possibility of being, in principle, refuted, a theory or hypothesis has no scientific content.

Although not all philosophers of science are Popperians, his work has had a dominant impact on how we think of science, and his is possibly the dominant view subscribed to by scientists in this latter part of the twentieth century[13]. As we noted earlier with Kuhn, history shows quite clearly that scientists have frequently not acted in the way Popper describes and, despite his claim that this is bad science, acting in this way has often advanced a scientific paradigm. Frequently scientists have ignored falsifications and, for Kuhn, in many cases they were correct to do so. In some ways, Popper's view is really one of how science should be carried out within the formal rules of logic, while Kuhn's account is how it is carried out in the real world, with all its imperfections. The contrast is between a rational construction (some would say reconstruction) and an historical one.

Critical rationalism implies that the methods of science are applicable to the area of health as well as natural science, and that the associated biological and social sciences provide the knowledge base for clinical practice. Within the health disciplines of the twentieth century, the dominant view has become that of health sciences as opposed to the healing arts. Historically, chiropractic has followed a similar path. The standard chiropractic curriculum provides as much education in basic science as that of medicine[14].

As noted in the previous chapter, contemporary chiropractic is highly involved in research – particularly in health services research but also, increasingly, in basic science. This has spawned a lively debate in the profession about whether the 'philosophy of chiropractic' can survive in the empiricist framework of science. This has led several writers to explore the use of more experiential models of research drawn from the social sciences such as phenomenology. However, this is less a rejection of critical rationalism or science than a plea for appropriate scientific models that can investigate and capture the notion of a holistic practice.

Experiential philosophies

Experiential philosophy has given rise to numerous paradigms that stand in stark contrast to those embraced by the natural sciences[15]. Many of these arose out of a critique of the reductionist, materialistic, deterministic paradigms, and their relevance for the social sciences.

The biomedical paradigm has been subjected to this same critique; in particular, its dualism. Within contemporary medicine Engel's[16] biopsychosocial paradigm, in which due attention is paid in illness to the psychological and social components of the patient's problems, is an expression of this same critique. Here, primacy is not given to biological factors and the physician must weigh the balance of all factors. Illness is seen in the full context of the patient's life.

Historically, this split between two major approaches to health has its roots in ancient Greek philosophy and two distinct schools of healing[17]. One, the Aesculapian philosophy, had as its central tenet a mechanistic view of health and illness, and adopted the investigative tools used for studying nature (what became the philosophy of science). It came to see diseases as arising from specific causes and giving rise to predictable diseases (and specific symptoms). The purpose of the practitioner was to seek the cause and the cure by treating the disease entity itself. The Hygeian philosophy of ancient Greece, in contrast, based on *vis medicatrix naturae*, rejected the separation of mind body and adopted a holistic approach to health. Here the role of the practitioner was to facilitate health, to help the natural healing of the body – 'in this view it is the patient who gets well and not the doctor who makes him well. Cure comes from within or not at all. Nor can health – any more than courage, integrity, or wisdom – be imparted by one person to another'[18]. It is interesting to note that Hippocrates, who provided the Hippocratic oath for modern medicine, belonged to the Hygeian school of thought.

The major philosophical underpinning for the alternative paradigms is that of phenomenology. At its simplest, phenomenology tries to understand the individual's experience of the world[19]. To do so, however, involves bringing subjectivity back into the picture. In phenomenology, the object and the perception of the object are inseparable. In health, it means that we should be concerned with understanding illness as it is lived[20]. Phenomenology arose as a reaction to the mind–body split of Descartes. It also was a way of acknowledging the importance and dignity of humans. Phenomenology conceptualizes human nature as based on responses to phenomenon as experienced subjectively by the individual. Individuals are seen as free-acting agents, who create the meanings of objects to which they respond. If we wish to know why they respond the way they do, we must capture these meanings. Behaviour in this view is not simply a response to externally applied forces, but is constructed in reaction to the attributed meanings that objects, events and illness have for the social actors themselves. This type of research is therefore known as grounded (grounded in the experience of the subject rather than the researcher), and it provides an alternative investigatory paradigm for chiropractic that is distinct from the positivist/empiricist one of natural science[21]. A range of research methods with a phenomeno-logical philosophical basis has developed, such as hermeneutics, symbolic interactionism, ethnomethodology and ethnography. All adopt essentially qualitative methods for investigating events. Their strength is that, in one way or another, they all acknowledge the importance of the perspective of the subjects/participants. For many authors, a phenomenological-based paradigm is essential for inves-tigating a holistic health practice[19,20,21,22].

From all these many philosophies, chiropractors have created a paradigm that embraces a philosophy of health and a philosophy of health care. Although chiropractors will individually differ, partic-ularly with regard to the metaphysical aspects of the paradigm, there is a reasonable degree of uniformity with regard to what is considered health and health care within the profession.

A philosophy of health

Historically, many commentators on chiropractic argued that what distinguished medicine from chiropractic was that the latter did not subscribe to the germ theory of disease. While this was clearly a distortion of chiropractic, even if it was true it would not lead to a dramatic distinction between the two paradigms. Since the germ theory is about the causes of disease, substituting another cause should not necessarily lead to a different health focus, although it might lead to quite different therapies. Both models could still fight the same health problems, simply using different therapies and giving different causal explanations. This is not in fact what happened. Chiropractic and medicine have largely focused on distinct health problems, and with quite different philosophies about health[23].

A discussion of the chiropractic approach to germs is instructive for understanding how both chiropractic and alternative health paradigms emerged in opposition to medicine. Palmer, like many of the alternative providers, reacted vigorously against the over-emphasis given to the germ theory of disease and the overuse of radical therapies derived as a result of the theory. In a sense, what Palmer challenged was the theory's ability to explain the distribution of disease. Why was it that two individuals occupying presumably, the same bacterially dangerous environment did not both succumb to germs? For Palmer, the only rational explanation was that there were differences in the ability of individuals to combat disease. Palmer concluded that the cause of disease was to be found within the person. If the body is functionally normal, it is able to resist germs and disease; therefore, when disease does occur, it does so because of a failure in the body's natural defence system (which Palmer termed dis-ease). He believed that, as long as the nervous system is intact and functioning normally, the body is able to combat disease naturally. The body is an integral unit and, as long as it maintains this integrity, it is capable of maintaining its own health. If chiropractors truly did not believe in germs, it would be difficult to explain why hygiene has been taught and practised within chiropractic colleges from the very beginning. Also, while chiropractic reacted to the over-emphasis on the germ therapy, it never opposed drug therapy for all problems; only the overuse and abuse of drug therapy. Chiropractic therefore did not deny the existence of germs, but made a distinction between exciting and predisposing causes. Disease occurs because of lowered resistance, which is the predisposing factor that allows germs (the exciting factor) to be effective. Diseases are therefore, in this paradigm, symptoms and not causes.

Chiropractic principles

Historically, chiropractors have expressed their philosophy of health as a set of principles, and most chiropractic colleges list 'Principles' as a dedicated course within the curriculum. Within these courses, the students are introduced to the metaphysics, dogma, philosophy, history, theory, central tenets, science and principles of chiroprac-tic[24]. To the author's knowledge, no other health profession has an equivalent course that is included almost without exception as a recognized course, although chiropractic colleges differ in what is always included. The purpose of the course is to establish the identity of chiropractic by introducing the history, battles, growth and possibilities of chiropractic. Sociologists would term these collectively the ideology of the chiropractic role. Ultimately, the principles are seen as the rationales for chiropractic. In the words of one college's historical calendar, 'this course is intended to create a form within which the student can accommodate all the disparate scientific data he {sic} will accumulate over the following years. It should give meaning to his labours, direction to his education, and value to his accomplishments'. It is in the area of principles that the colleges will articulate their particular philosophy of chiropractic. Traditionally, it is in this area that a college will identify itself as either a straight or mixed college.

The number of identified principles will vary greatly. Stephenson (1948) listed 33 principles he thought characterized Palmer's chiropractic (27 of which make a direct reference to innate intelligence)[25]. B. J. Palmer himself endorsed Stephenson's compilation of the principles. There are at least five basic principles that chiropractors accept, and these were outlined by the Palmers and articulated by Forster in 1923[27]. These are:

1   Subluxations, particularly of the vertebrae, do occur

2   Such subluxations may cause impingement on the contents of the intervertebral foramen

3   As a result, the irritability of the corresponding segment of the spinal cord and its connecting spinal and autonomic nerves is reduced, and the conduction of the nerves is impaired

4   Certain parts of the organism are deprived of their innervation and become either dis-eased or prone to dis-ease

5   Adjustment of a subluxation removes the impingement and restores innervation to the diseased parts, thereby rehabilitating them[26].

Within chiropractic, the epochal event was the first chiropractic adjustment given by D. D. Palmer in 1895 (although the veracity of this date has now been challenged). This was a specific adjustment given to an individual who was deaf, which restored his hearing. While Palmer claimed that this was a specific adjustment, the results of which were what he had intended, and that he had the theory and principles prior to this event, many writers have challenged this interpretation, suggesting that Palmer may not initially have understood what he had done. Whatever the truth about the actual event, as an anecdote it contains all the elements that, when elaborated, result in the chiropractic paradigm. A spinal lesion was corrected using the hand, and restored normal functioning to a structure far removed from the spine. The problem therefore was one of structural pathology that was reversible, and was biomechanical with neurophysiological impact. Along with the therapeutic event, a theoretical explanation was given (subluxation) and a metaphysic was developed (the innate). It should be noted that not all chiropractors subscribe to the principles developed by the Palmers; nor did they historically. Many early followers of Palmer broke away to develop their own schools and philosophies. One such group was termed the rational alternative[27], and split over the increasing role of metaphysical beliefs in chiropractic, which they saw as a distortion of D. D. Palmer's original emphasis on the science of chiropractic.

More recently, Winterstein[28] has articulated 11 principles while Phillips and colleagues[3] have isolated four key principles. While there is therefore some variance in the number of principles, the four principles identified by the latter constitute a core set in that they are embraced by all the systems, although others expand the number. The four principles are:

1   Health is the natural state of individuals, and any departure from this state represents a failure of the individual to adapt to the internal and external environment, or the result of adverse adaptation. The innate tendency of the body is to restore and maintain health and this is accomplished by (compensating) homeostatic mechanisms, reparative processes and adaptive responses to genetic and acquired limitations.

2   Health is an expression of biological, psychological, social and spiritual factors, and disease and illness is multi-causal. This is a holistic philosophy of health.

3   Optimal health is unique for any individual. It involves enabling persons to realistically fulfil their biological, human, and social potentials. This also implies individual responsibility for health. The chiropractor is simply the facilitator and, through co-operation with the patient, patient education and

adherence, they together achieve health for the patient. Health also implies a belief in healthy living (good nutrition, constructive exercise, stress management and good posture).

 The structure and functioning of the neuromusculoskeletal system is central to the maintenance of good health and the combating of disease. The functioning of the musculoskeletal system is integrated with neurological function, and is expressed by the various regulatory systems of the body.

These four principles do not specifically refer to the concept of subluxation, although they would clearly allow for its inclusion. The chiropractic profession is split over this issue. One group sees subluxation as an important historical concept used by Palmer and chiropractic to develop a theoretical explanation for the lesion being treated. This school of thought feels it has outlived its usefulness in contemporary chiropractic, having failed to be substantiated by research and providing little in the way of generating new research. A second group feels just as strongly that the concept of subluxation is the *raison d'être* of chiropractic practice. In the middle is a third group, who have proposed a variant called the subluxation complex paradigm as an heuristic device for integrating the complex knowledge surrounding the adjustment and the lesion being adjusted. Although much is made in the profession over this conflict, from a scholarly point of view it is really a difference over a theoretical explanation that in other fields would be seen as a natural part of the discipline. However, as with most things in chiropractic, it has taken on doctrinal significance, with various groups adopting very dogmatic positions *vis-à-vis* the issue.

Summary

A key element of this philosophy of health is the distinction made between health and disease, whereby health is not seen simply as the absence of disease – the traditional stance of medicine. This approach also makes a distinction between disease and illness; whereas the former refers to pathology, the latter refers to the social, cultural and psychological expression of disease. All illness has a subjective component, which may be more debilitating than the disease. The concept of illness draws attention to the sick role the individual plays. Under this philosophy of health the role of the provider is to treat the illness, and not simply the underlying pathology.

A philosophy of health care

From the above philosophy of health, it is possible to derive a philosophy of health care. In some ways this is deducible from the above principles or, at the very least, is logically consistent with them. To the extent that illness is multifactorial, the need is for a form of health care that embraces a holistic approach. In this philosophy, the concept of the health-care provider is distinct. The health-care provider is involved in natural healing of the total patient, and is seen primarily as a facilitator and an educator. Furthermore, the emphasis is on caring as opposed to simply treatment. Briefly, this type of provider is expected to:

❑ be holistic in focus (non-reductionistic)
❑ be humanistic, treating the patient as an equal and reinforcing the dignity of the patient in settings that are not alienating and impersonal
❑ use natural therapies
❑ be therapeutically conservative, using the least intervention possible
❑ use a low level of technology and a high level of personal involvement and individualized care regimens
❑ be caring and kind.

The latter captures an idea expressed by Andrew Still, the founder of osteopathy, that there are two ways to make a reputation; you can be clever or kind[29].

For Vernon[30], characteristics of a neuromusculoskeletal holistic provider are:

❑ concern for the illness of the patient
❑ an emphasis on ambulatory care, maintaining and achieving movement in the structures in the lower back and pelvis, and thereby in the patient as a whole
❑ a rational explanation to patients to reduce distress

❏ an emphasis on recovery of full function, rather than rest and symptomatic relief (this requires the active presence and impact of the health-care giver in the process of functional recovery)
❏ being active and empathetic, as opposed to an aloof practitioner.

The chiropractor is a primary contact health-care provider (the patient may access them directly) and, according to some authors, provide primary care (this claim will be explored more fully in the following chapter). For the most part, their focus is on 'functional pathology', not in the sense of a diseased pathology, but in the sense of disruptions to the neuromusculoskeletal system. Functional pathology is being used here metaphorically. Around this primary focus, chiropractors have developed a 'wellness' paradigm that is involved in extensive lifestyle counselling in such areas as stress, posture, exercise, nutrition, ergonomics, etc. If we think historically, health care in this century has focused on treatment of disease (medicine), preventive programmes (public health), health promotion (health education) and, only recently, health enhancement. It is in this last area that chiropractic and alternative health care have been particularly focused; where the point of the intervention is not simply to solve the current health problem, but to address the total health of the patient.

Implications

One of the implications of the chiropractic philosophy of health and the crucial role of the individuals in their own health is that the treatment paradigm has been overly patient-oriented, a patient-centred paradigm[8]. This has also been a matter of pragmatics since, like all alternative providers in a culture where the traditional route for illness is medicine, chiropractors have been required to pay attention both to patient's needs and to getting results. Patients in alternative health care have invariably used other forms of care first and, failing to get results, have turned elsewhere. Gatterman[8] has isolated six features of a patient-centred paradigm in chiropractic:

1   Recognition and facilitation of the inherent healing capacity of the person

2   Recognition that care should ideally focus on the total person

③ Acknowledgment and respect for the patient's values and beliefs, and health-care needs and expectations

④ Promotion of the patient's health through a preference for drugless, minimally invasive and conservative care where indicated

⑤ A proactive approach that encourages patients to take responsibility for their health

⑥ The patient and the patient-centred practitioner act as partners in decision making, emphasizing clinically and economically effective care, based on predictable delivery, documentable outcome and overall quality.

Conclusion

This chapter began with the claim that chiropractic philosophy was a misnomer, but that there could be a viable philosophy of chiropractic. However, the term is misnomer in another sense. Chiropractic does not contain a single philosophy, but is comprised of several major philosophies, at the very least those of vitalism, holism, naturalism, therapeutic conservatism, humanism and critical rationalism. We also noted that a strong philosophy of chiropractic would help to answer important questions such as: What is the nature and purpose of chiropractic? What kinds of concepts populate chiropractic, and how do they explain disease, illness, health, treatment and cure? What kind of science is chiropractic? What is the nature of the clinical art of chiropractic? What kind of values does chiropractic embrace? In exploring the philosophy of chiropractic in this chapter, we have begun to answer these questions. Chiropractic gave rise to a particular philosophy of health, and a particular philosophy of health care. The former is not unique to chiropractic, and is widely shared by such other alternative health care as homeopathy, naturopathy and osteopathy (to name only those forms that were adopted or developed in North America at the same time as chiropractic). The latter, however, with its emphasis on the role of the treatment of the neuromusculoskeletal system, begins to focus more specifically on the uniqueness of chiropractic. Even here, however, osteopathy would appear to differ, primarily with regard to a theoretical difference. Historically, the emphasis in osteopathy was on the circulatory system and the impact of the osteopathic lesion ('subluxation' in chiropractic terms) on the circulatory system, as opposed to the impact on the neural system proposed by chiropractic. They followed quite distinct pathways for professional acceptance but, to an outside observer, the differences in terms of philosophy are less than the similarities. Ultimately, the philosophy of chiropractic has real impact, that is, it is something more than rhetoric, if we can show that, in practice, it leads to a discernible difference that is both considered important by the patients and has distinct therapeutic outcomes. The next chapter will explore this issue. The following, however, should already be clear:

1   Philosophical issues are inextricably involved in the practice of chiropractic

2   Much of the intellectual history of chiropractic has been around these issues

3   The so-called chiropractic wars internal to the profession have been over the same issues

4   Those external to the profession have had great difficulty in understanding the nature and importance of these philosophical issues

5   These same issues have often led the profession to be ridiculed by those opposed to chiropractic

6   These same issues also characterize, in one form or another, the other alternative health-care providers.

References

[1] Ladd, J. (1979). Philosophy of medicine. In *Changing Values in Medicine* (E. J. Cassell and M. Sigler, eds), pp. 205–16. University Publishers of America.
[2] Coulter, I. D. (1991). An institutional philosophy of chiropractic. *Chiropr. J. Aust.*, **21(4)**, 136–41.
[3] Phillips R. B., Coulter, I. D., Adams, A. *et al.* (1994). A contemporary philosophy of chiropractic for the Los Angeles College of Chiropractic. *J. Chiropr. Human.*, **4**, 20–25.

[4] Bryner, P. (1987). Isn't it time to abandon anachronistic terminology? *J. Aust. Chiropr. Ass.*, **17**, 53–9.

[5] Koch, D. (1996). Has vitalism been a help or a hindrance to the science and art of chiropractic? *J. Chiropr. Human.*, **6(1)**, 18–22.

[6] Lowenberg, J. S. (1989). *Caring and Responsibility.* University of Pennsylvania.

[7] Gordon, J. S. (1980). The paradigm of holistic medicine. In *Health for the Whole Person* (A. C. Hastings, J. Fadiman and J. S. Gordon, eds), pp. 16–22. Westview Press.

[8] Gatterman, M. I. (1995). A Patient-centered paradigm: a model for chiropractic education and research. *J. Alt. Compl. Med.*, **1(4)**, 371–86.

[9] Korr, I. M. (1991). Osteopathic research: the needed paradigm shift. *J. Am. Osteopath. Ass.*, **91**, 160–71.

[10] Jamison, J. R. (1996). Psychoneuroendoimmunology: the biological basis of the placebo phenomenon. *J. Manipul. Physiol. Ther.*, **19(7)**, 484–7.

[11] Palmer, D. D. (1910). *The Science, Art and Philosophy of Chiropractic.* Portland Printing House.

[12] Popper, K. R. (1969*). Conjectures and Refutations. The Growth of Scientific Knowledge.* Routledge and Kegan Paul.

[13] Radnitzky, G. (1968). *Contemporary Schools of Metascience. Anglo-Saxon Schools of Metascience. Continental Schools of Metascience.* Henry Regnery Company.

[14] Coulter, I. D., Adams, A., Coogan, P. *et al.* (1998). A comparative study of chiropractic and medical education. *Alt. Ther. Health Med.*, **4(5)**, 64–75.

[15] Beckman, J., Fernandez, C. and Coulter, I. D. (1995). A systems model of health care: a proposal. *J. Manipul. Physiol. Ther.*, **19(3)**, 208–15.

[16] Engel, G. L. (1977). The need for a new medical model: a challenge for biomedicine. *Science* **196**, 129–36.

[17] Coulter, I. D. (1983). Chiropractic and medical education. A contrast in models of health and illness. *J. Can. Chiropr. Ass.*, **27(4)**, 151–8.

[18] Korr, I. M. and Ogilvie, C. D. (1987). Health orientation in medical education, United States: the Texas College of Osteopathic Medicine. *Prevent. Med.*, **10**, 710–18.

[19] O'Malley, J. N. (1995). Toward a reconstruction of the philosophy of chiropractic. *J. Manipul. Physiol. Ther.*, **18(5)**, 285–92.

[20] Kleynhans, A. M. (1991). Developing philosophy in chiropractic. *Chiropr. J. Aust.*, **21(4)**, 161–7.

[21] Coulter, I. D. (1993). Alternative philosophical and investigatory paradigms for chiropractic. *J. Manipul. Physiol. Ther.*, **6(3)**, 419–25.

[22] Jamison, J. R. (1997). An interactive model of chiropractic practice: reconstructing clinical reality. *J. Manipul. Physiol. Ther.*, **20(4)**, 382–8.

[23] Coulter, I. D. (1981) The chiropractic curriculum: a problem of integration. *J. Manipul. Physiol. Ther.*, **4(3)**, 147–54.

[24] Stephenson, R.W. (1948). *Chiropractic.* Davenport, Palmer School of Chiropractic.

[25] Coulter, I. D. (1990). The chiropractic paradigm. *J. Manipul. Physiol. Ther.*, **13(5)**, 279–87.

[26] Forster, A. C. (1923) *Principles and Practice of Chiropractic*. National Publishing Association.

[27] Beideman, R. P. (1983). Seeking the rational alternative: the National College of Chiropractic from 1906 to 1982. *Chiropr. Hist.*, **3(1)**, 17–22.

[28] Winterstein, J. W. (1994). Philosophy of chiropractic: a contemporary perspective (Parts 1 and 2). *Am. Chiropr. Ass. J.*, **May**, 28–36, 64–71.

[29] Ward, R. C. (1977) Osteopathic theory: a strategy for curriculum integration. *J. Am. Osteopath. Ass.*, **76**, 414–22.

[30] Vernon, H. (1991). A model for incorporating the illness behavior model in the management of low back pain patients. *J. Manipul. Physiol. Ther.*, **14(6)**, 379–89.

5 The clinical art of chiropractic

Although the therapies of chiropractic are not used exclusively in chiropractic, the health problems presented to the chiropractor are not unique and the philosophy of chiropractic shares much in common with other alternative providers, chiropractors have been able to create a practice that patients experience as unique and value highly. They have also been able to create an independent and unique profession that has not only survived but flourished for over 100 years. Perhaps the uniqueness lies not in any single element but in the constellation of the elements experienced in the health encounter by the patient, in the clinical art of chiropractic. The end result is that the patients do experience chiropractic as unique, and that chiropractic has established a unique role within the health-care system. Patients do not confuse chiropractors with their other providers, and society generally clearly distinguishes chiropractic within the health-care system as distinct and separate from other health-care providers. This is no mean achievement, and examination of it might also illuminate why 40 per cent of the population is attracted to, and continues to use, alternative health care. This chapter will examine what is known about the chiropractic health encounter and the role of the chiropractor within the broader health-care system.

The chiropractic health encounter

It is clear from studies looking at the epidemiology of chiropractic patients that the overwhelming majority of patients present for a narrow range of conditions. Three conditions account for around 70 per cent of the conditions presented (lower back is the most common, followed by face/neck pain, followed by mid back pain)[1]. National surveys in the United States[2] also indicate that spinal subluxation/joint dysfunction and headaches are the conditions routinely seen. In addition, conditions listed as frequently seen are overwhelmingly neuromuscoloskeletal in origin and, furthermore, manipulation/adjustment is the most frequently performed and billed service by chiropractors[3]. Looking at these statistics, chiropractic appears to be largely dominated by one mode of therapy (adjustments) and focused on a very narrow range of health problems.

Such social epidemiology, however, gives no indication about the nature of the health encounter or the type of care delivered. Those studies that have used an observational method to study the health encounter present a view about chiropractic that stands in marked contrast to the epidemiology of chiropractic practice. Unfortunately, to date few such studies exist. Four such studies are discussed below.

Kelner et al., 1980

The study by Kelner and colleagues[4] remains the most extensive study of this type conducted. It is also unique in the extent to which it combined quantitative and qualitative data within the same study. The study involved an extensive field study of chiropractic practice and patients. A random sample of one in five Canadian chiropractors, stratified for rural and urban, was surveyed, giving a total of 349 chiropractors. From this group, 70 practices were randomly chosen for further in-depth interviews with the chiropractors, an ethnographic observation study of the clinics over a single day, and interviews with 10 randomly chosen patients in each clinic on each day. Wherever possible, the patient interviewed was also observed during the encounter with the chiropractor. The total patient sample was 658. In addition, one participant observation case study was conducted where a researcher was enrolled as a patient for 6 months.

From these multiple sources, the researchers constructed a model of the healing encounter. The study showed that, despite what appears to be a very limited scope in terms of epidemiology, around these conditions the chiropractor has constructed a broad-based health encounter. The researchers concluded, therefore, that the chiropractic role is not confined to intervention through manipulation, even if the bulk of effort is in this direction. The chiropractor 'is also involved, with the patient's co-operation, in preventing occurrences of health problems, either through continuing chiropractic treatment or by effecting changes in the patient's behavior'[4]. The authors concluded that chiropractors are involved in holistic care; that is, care that goes beyond the immediate presented problem to total management, including advice on nutrition, posture, exercise, stress management, etc. The chiropractor expands the care into the areas of prevention, maintenance, and enhancement. It is conservative care, in the sense that it uses low-level technology for the most part and adjustment with few, if any, side effects. The care is readily available, in that chiropractors tended to practise at times and in locations convenient for the patients. It was noted that, for the most part, chiropractic care is immediate, beginning with the first visit (there is no prolonged testing or waiting for results), and it frequently offers immediate relief and early restoration of functioning. The researchers noted observing numerous instances of 'miraculous' relief for individuals presenting with severe back pain. It also provides personal care, in that each patient requires an individual orientation because they differ in size, weight, type of problem and difficulty in adjusting. Although technically patients may receive the same type of adjustment (for example, a cervical adjustment), the variation in how it is delivered may be vast.

The care also appeared intelligible; that is, the care is accompanied by explanations that the patients feel they understand and in terms and a language that is comprehensible to them. Chiropractic care also involves making the patients aware of their personal responsibility for their own health. To a high degree, the care is co-operative care, with the patients as partners.

Coulehan, 1985

A study by Coulehan[5], although much smaller in scope (10 chiropractors), reported a health encounter very similar to the above. His chiropractic health encounter has four major features. The first is that the chiropractor brings to the encounter a belief system with not only a positive regard for the patient and genuineness ('the ability to be oneself in the relationship without hiding behind a role or façade'[5]), but also a positive view that what they do helps the patient. Where the medical practitioner sees back problems as difficult and uncertain, the chiropractor sees them as solvable. Coulehan calls this 'the faith that heals'. The second feature is explanations that are understandable to the patient and both mechanical and holistic. The former concepts are ones acceptable in a rationalistic society, and the latter appeal to the patient's sense that the person is not subtracted from the encounter. Chiropractic also stresses a positive dynamic, drug-free view of health – 'the net effect is a logical set of beliefs which appeal to common sense, use scientific terminology, yet promote a natural, non-invasive, holistic approach rather than a medical approach ...'[5]. Third, chiropractors do something to the patient rather than simply talk or write prescriptions. This involves extensive laying on of hands, which attends to bodily pain, and touching. The fourth component of the encounter is a plan 'that requires patient commitment and co-operation'[5]. This may include a programme of exercise, nutritional counselling, stress management techniques and behavioural change. Coulehan[5] concludes that 'chiropractic care, as opposed to spinal adjustment as an isolated treatment, must be viewed as a process or interaction ...'.

Jamison, 1993

A third observation study[6] also involved interviews with practitioners (34), and the viewing of patient files. This study concluded that, while the chiropractors were providing holistic care, there were three ideal types that sometimes operated simultaneously within the doctor–patient relationship. The care involved manual, emotional, and psycho-social contact. It was co-operative, focused on the wellbeing of the patient, used a low level of technology, focused on objective, subjective and effective data, was directed at understanding the whole person and was personalized. The three ideal types (paradigms) identified were biomechanical, conventional holism and alternate holism. The first stresses the body as a machine, the second stresses the multifactorial nature of health care, and the last focuses on a vitalistic version of holism. Like Coulehan, Jamison found that, when explaining to the patients, the chiropractors tend to use rationalistic, reductionist concepts of biomechanics. However, if the focus is on the chiropractors' understandings and expectations (the cognitive commitment), then it is clearly holistic. Furthermore, this is reflected both in the nature of the doctor–patient relationship and, in particular, in the total discourse between the two. The objective for the chiropractor is the total wellbeing of the patient, even if the initial focus is manipulation of a specific lesion. Considering the presenting symptoms, and the application of therapy therefore, the encounter resembles that of a reductionist, non-holistic practitioner. This, however, misses the essence of the encounter. It is therapy delivered within a much broader paradigm.

In terms of the encounter, the study concluded that every consultation with the chiropractor involved the establishment or reinforcement of a personal relationship between the chiropractor and the patient. This was accomplished by the interest shown by the chiropractor both in the patient's problem and in the impact it was having. It was reinforced by an interest shown in friends, the family, community and the social activities of the patient, and these were often linked to conversations and inquiries from the previous visit, giving continuity to the interest. It was often reinforced by the fact that other family members used the same chiropractor. Second, the patient and the provider shared in a dialogue about the diagnosis, the current status, progress achieved and the therapy. In this way, the patient and the chiropractor tended to share common definitions of the therapeutic reality. Again, this study found that the patients had a high level of understanding (86 per cent expected to understand their condition better after the visit) and that the explanations reduced their uncertainty. Overwhelmingly, the patients found the take-home advice helpful and understandable, and 91 per cent felt they were more confident about coping after seeing the chiropractor. Last but not least, the study found that both verbal and non-verbal communication was operating in the encounter, and that both contributed to the bonding between the patient and the provider. Pain, soreness and tenderness are frequently associated symptoms with nueromusculoskeletal problems, and the chiropractors' ability manually to elicit verbal and non-verbal responses such as grimaces, grunts and yelps provided useful feedback for the chiropractor and confirmation for the patients that their pain was being focused on.

Jamison, 1997

In another study, Jamison[7] also examined the co-operative nature of chiropractic care. She found that the chiropractors expected patients to play a role in their health management, and that the patients were aware of this. Jamison also noted that, through the use of explanations and patient education, the chiropractors were empowering the patients to make decisions and have personal control over their health status[8].

Summary

The results of these studies therefore reflect a much broader scope of practice for chiropractic than is suggested by the epidemiology of the patient complaints and the dominance of manipulation/adjustment as a therapy. Surveys in the United States[2] have indicated that two-thirds of chiropractors use 12 major non-adjustive techniques (for example, 96 per cent use exercise, 84 per cent use nutritional counselling, 73 per cent use electrical stimulation and 73 per cent use massage). The above studies also suggest that it is within the full health encounter that the essence of chiropractic is experienced by the patient. The question, therefore, is how this role might be captured within contemporary philosophy of health. One possible way of examining this encounter is to look at it within the context of a wellness practitioner.

The chiropractor as a wellness practitioner

The notion of a wellness practitioner[9,10,11], and in fact the wellness movement, has arisen from a critique of the current health-care system and the doctor–patient relationship. In essence, the critics have argued that we do not have a *health*-care system but a *sick*-care system, the focus of which is on disease (the physiological expression) and illness (the social expression) rather than on health as such. This critique[12] has focused extensively on biomedicine, and includes the following:

❑ An historical re-evaluation of the contribution of medicine to health
❑ The changing epidemiology of illnesses, from infections to behaviour-induced illness
❑ The discovery of iatrogenic illness
❑ The recognition of the importance of psychosomatic illness
❑ The recognition of the role of social and historical factors on health
❑ Studies of inequities in health care and the unequal burden of illness
❑ A consumer critique
❑ A humanist critique focusing on the bureaucracy and impersonality of contemporary medicine
❑ Cross-cultural studies
❑ The economic critique of escalating costs.

This state of affairs has many causes, but for many critics the main causes are as follows:

❑ Medicine embracing the ideology of scientism
❑ The biologizing of illness
❑ The reduction of illness to specific causes
❑ The dualism embraced between mind and body
❑ The elevation of pathology/anatomy as the basis for diagnosis and intervention
❑ The loss of the traditional 'whole person' perspective.

Wellness practitioners are conceived as the antithesis of current medical practitioners. They are holistic (non-reductionist), humanistic, naturalistic (use natural remedies); conservative (the least therapy being the best therapy), egalitarian, caring, and use a low level of technology. An important element of the wellness movement is that health is something other than simply the absence of disease.

> Wellness is more than a concept. It is a way of life, an integrated enjoyable approach to living that emphasizes the importance of achieving harmony in all parts of the person; mind, body, spirit. It is a lifestyle that creates the greatest potential for personal wellbeing. More than the absence of illness, it is a balance among all the aspects of the person.
>
> Coulter[13]

Disease refers to a disordered biology. The subjective experience of this, and the behaviour associated with it, is illness (referred to by sociologists as 'the sick role'). The absence of disease has traditionally been conceived as health. In a wellness paradigm, however, there is the recognition that health involves much more than the absence of disease, and that health care should therefore involve more than the treatment of disease. It also posits that treatment is distinguishable from care. In a wellness paradigm, health care involves both treatment therapies (such as manipulation) and also a whole range of activities aimed at overall health 'care' of the individual, such as identifying illness behaviour, restorative care, health promotion, health enhancement through lifestyle counselling, and behaviour modification. As noted earlier, chiropractic, by using a wide range of natural and conservative therapies, is directed towards the restoration and enhancement of health. Health in a wellness paradigm is viewed in terms of human potential.

> A person's optimum state of health is equivalent to the state of the set of conditions which fulfil his or her realistic chosen and biological potentials. Some of these conditions are of the highest importance for all people. Others are variable, dependent upon individual abilities and circumstances.
>
> Seedhouse[14]

Philosophy of wellness

In the last chapter, four principles were described to characterize the chiropractic philosophy of health[15]. These same principles are also a philosophy of wellness. To reiterate:

1. Health is the natural state of the individual, and the natural tendency of the body is to maintain or restore that health

2. Health is an expression of biological, psychological, social and spiritual factors, and disease and illness is multicausal

3. Optimal health is unique for any single individual, and the individual also bears some responsibility for their health – the practitioner is simply a facilitator of health

There is a fundamental and central role for the structure and function of the neuromusculoskeletal system in the maintenance of good health and combating disease.

Vernon[16] has offered a clear model for what such a perspective would mean in chiropractic practice. He argues that chiropractic's success in treating low back pain may have more to do with its success with the illness behaviour than with the 'disease'. That is, the success of chiropractic care may have more to do with the clinical art than the manipulative therapy. He develops a theoretical framework that distinguishes disease and illness, treatment and care in terms of its practical application; that is, what a provider will do in practice following such a paradigm. Under the paradigm, Vernon suggests a radical reshaping of the doctor–patient relationship and their roles:

> The physician will be a facilitator, enabling patients to cope with their problems, while, for the patient, a new role of active sharing of the responsibility for his/her own progress will emerge. The clinical paradigm will thus shift from treatment to care.
>
> Vernon[16]

This practice paradigm involves a management pathway comprised of four stages; reduction of pain, recovery of function, rehabilitation and reinforcement. For each stage, the clinical objectives include both the *treatment* and the *illness*. For example, in Stage I (reduction of pain), the treatment objectives for the clinic include recommending rest, ice/heat therapy, modalities, low-force manual soft tissue therapeutics and low-force or passive mobilizing to the patient's tolerance. Home treatment includes effective bed rest, ice/heat applications, supports and useful lifestyle modifications. On the illness behaviour side, his clinical objectives include reduction of anxiety and activation of patient co-operation. Vernon also identifies the typical abnormal behaviours that are associated with low back pain, such as excessive antalgia, limping, vocalizations, uncontrolled and ineffective down-time, poor self help, loss of control of lifestyle, excessive self-medication, poor help-seeking behaviour and acting out within the family unit. Strategies recommended for improving illness behaviour include advice regarding effective rest and down-time, advice regarding effective self help, and establishing control of lifestyle and help-seeking as a major objective for the patient. Vernon lays out the same format for each of the four stages of management. This is a clinical articulation of a chiropractic wellness paradigm.

Left unanswered is whether an adjustment as such has a unique role in wellness care over and above its role as treatment therapy. Balduc[17] has attempted to identify the unique role of the adjustment by focusing on the anatomical and physiological mechanisms that promote wellness:

> The central feature of this wellness knowledge is the appreciation that the nervous system plays a prominent role in total body (holistic) physiology.
>
> Balduc[17]

From a wellness point of view, the body is equipped with an integrative physiology. For Balduc, subluxation represents a challenge to the integrity of this system, and its removal a restoration of that integrity. Jamison[18] also proposes a similar self-organizing biological system with the adjustment triggering the rule-governed process, which then initiates the process of wellness. The treatment of a single subluxation at one level has repercussions throughout the system, and it is this that affects the total system. A structural intervention therefore has global effects:

> The goal of chiropractic consultation, rather than being documentation of a particular diagnostic entity, is correction of a dysfunction with the relief of pain, restoration of function and enhancement of wellbeing.
>
> Jamison[18]

A key part of Jamison's work has been to articulate the role of the chiropractor in health promotion as a primary contact provider[19].

The chiropractor as a primary health-care provider

Initially, primary health care was simply a term denoting the point at which the patient enters the health-care system and, clearly, chiropractic is a point of entry. However, this has come to be termed 'primary contact', and means simply that a patient may go directly to a provider (as in the case of a dentist, for example). There are three broad perspectives, as outlined by Kranz[20], for viewing primary care in the health-care system; a social/societal perspective, a provider/physician perspective and a lay-patient/consumer perspective.

The social/societal perspective

The social/societal perspective includes not only the normal delivery system (doctors, nurses, hospitals, etc.) but also the environmental, social/welfare, economic and personal health-care factors, etc. This perspective is the one adopted by the World Health Organization (WHO). Here, the total social and environmental context is considered an integral part of primary health care and, under this definition, all providers would be considered limited primary care since none could deliver all the services needed.

The provider/physician perspective

For Kranz, the provider/physician perspective focuses on a personal health-care subset. This is commonly divided into primary (entry level), secondary (ambulatory services of a specialist nature) and tertiary (the medical hospital centre) levels. The primary level consists of providers who are generally concerned with acute, chronic, frequently occurring conditions that require minimal care. This is the level usually identified as primary care. However, there is much debate concerning how separate the three levels are (some hospitals provide primary care). It is also under contention whether primary care can only be given by a medical practitioner (or should simply be supervised and monitored by them), whether the care is illness or health care, and whether it is crisis, preventive and/or public health care.

The lay-patient/consumer perspective

The lay-patient/consumer perspective sees primary care as care that is accessible, affordable, given by a constant practitioner who knows the patient and that they can trust, and who can deal with a broad range of needs. For most people in Western culture, this is the family medical physician.

The professional perspective

For the most part, it has been the perspective of the professionals that has dominated primary care. Kranz surveyed health providers (and their associations) to obtain those attributes they thought were essential for quality primary care. The general consensus was that primary care:

- ❑ provides for the patients general health-care needs
- ❑ involves direct contact – the primary practitioner serves as the point-of-entry into the health-care system
- ❑ is accessible care – the providers are available and attainable 24 hours a day if required
- ❑ is acceptable – primary care provides care that is personal, individualist and acceptable to the patient and the provider of the care
- ❑ is accountable – the providers are responsible for the care they render, holding themselves accountable to a recognized standard of care
- ❑ includes education and counselling – primary providers teach patients, communities and societies about proper health and illness care
- ❑ involves co-ordination of care – primary providers must be able to co-ordinate the patient's care with other providers and specialists, communicate with the provider, and integrate all the facets of the care
- ❑ is continuous – primary providers give continuous, on-going health care
- ❑ is comprehensive – primary providers should be a source of the majority of services that supply a full range of services and a broad scope of treatment for a wide variety of frequent illnesses
- ❑ provides essential or basic care to the patient – this is care that is deemed necessary and desirable for the wellbeing of the patient and the community.

Kranz concludes that:

Primary care therefore would be care that provides for the general health needs of the patient; is a first or direct contact service; provides an assessment of health; is accessible to those who need it; is acceptable to the consumer of health-care services; is accountable; provides education and counselling; provides co-ordinated, continuous, comprehensive and essential care.

Kranz[20]

Is chiropractic primary health care?

If the WHO definition of primary care is accepted, neither chiropractic nor medicine would constitute primary health care. Wardwell concluded that the chiropractor is not a primary health-care provider:

Although they are not primary care providers, limited medical practitioners are 'portal of entry' to the health-care system, since they are the point of first contact to patients who have not undergone a medical diagnosis.

Wardwell[21]

For Kranz[20], chiropractic is primary contact and provides assessment (even if there is debate whether this is a full differential diagnosis). With regard to the criteria of accessible, acceptable, accountable, continuous and co-ordinated counselling, Kranz concludes that no data exist to substantiate chiropractic's claim to these. However, if we compare the results above from studies on the chiropractic health encounter the descriptions of chiropractic practice, they clearly have elements similar to those of the primary provider. For Kranz, the most troubling criteria for chiropractic are those of comprehensiveness and essential care. He concludes that chiropractic does not provide comprehensive care. In terms of essential care, he notes that the conditions chiropractors deal with are seldom life threatening, and that whole parts of the globe survive without any chiropractors whatsoever. Furthermore, the data on chiropractic utilization shows that chiropractors, in the main, are used for a limited range of health problems.

However, if we take the concept of wellness practitioner (as outlined above), we can distinguish two types of practitioner: an illness practitioner focused largely on disease (pathology) and trauma (injury), and another focused on wellness. This is not to suggest that the focus is exclusively one or the other. Clearly, illness practitioners also focus on prevention just as wellness practitioners must also be concerned about pathology; however, it does suggest that the thrust of the care is in different areas. The question then arises of whether the two practitioners provide primary health care but in different arenas.

Although chiropractic seems to have some of the attributes of primary practitioners, and virtually all those of the wellness practitioner, it does not claim to be comprehensive for illness care. However, with respect to wellness care (health care), a case can be made that chiropractic is (or is potentially) more comprehensive than medicine, especially with regard to such things as nutrition, posture, exercise, weight control, etc. Chiropractic does not compete with regard to serious pathology or trauma[22].

A study conducted by the Foundation for Chiropractic Education and Research (FCER)[23] examined the role of the chiropractor as a primary care provider in rural areas. Although based on the self reports of 260 chiropractors, and using the AMA's definition of primary care, the study found that 48 per cent of the chiropractors in areas of 1–10 000 inhabitants reported that 75–100 per cent of their patients used them as primary contact providers. The percentage was also highest in the most rural areas. In terms of providing services thought to be related to primary care, 97 per cent of the chiropractors took a history; most conducted diagnostic tests (palpation 100 per cent, auscultation 77 per cent, percussion 80 per cent, observation 99 per cent); and all were extensively involved in providing 'wellness' care (100 per cent provided guidance on exercise, 94 per cent counselled on lifestyle modification and 88 per cent offered nutritional advice). With regard to accessibility, 71 per cent referred patients to other providers when they were unavailable, 67 per cent left an emergency number and 45 per cent employed an answering service. Although no task analysis was performed, the results would suggest that some aspects of primary care may be provided, at least in rural areas, by chiropractors[23].

The question of whether or not chiropractic constitutes primary health care[24] has extensive policy ramifications. Historically, chiropractic did perceive itself as a broad-based health paradigm and not simply as a method of spinal adjustment with a focus on neuromusculoskeletal problems. However, the profession has been split politically over what this means in terms of the scope of practice and the therapies and modalities to be used in practice. The Council on Chiropractic Education (CCE) quite clearly sees its mission in terms of preparing a primary practitioner. Under *Mission and Goals*, the standards state that the purpose of a chiropractic education is:

> The preparation of the doctor of chiropractic as a *primary health-care provider*, as a portal of entry to the health-care delivery system, well educated to diagnose, to care for the human body, to understand and relate fundamental scientific education, and to consult with, or refer to, other health-care providers.
>
> CCE[25] (italics added)

The *Guidelines for Chiropractic Quality Assurance and Practice Parameters* (the result of a consensus development process, and referred to in chiropractic as the *Mercy Document*[26]), although not explicitly stating chiropractic as primary care, imply in the chapter on Collaborative Care, that chiropractic is primary. The chapter begins, 'All patients of all primary care health providers have the right to expect health-care services at the highest level of quality'. The chapter then deals with the guidelines for achieving this in chiropractic. Furthermore, its definition of a primary care doctor is[26]:

(1) any health-care provider capable of providing first level contact and intake into the health delivery system (portal-of-entry provider)
(2) any health-care provider licensed to receive patient contact in the absence of physician referral.

Such a definition would appear to include chiropractic.

The chiropractor as a specialist

Both within chiropractic and externally, there is a contrary view of chiropractic that sees the chiropractor either as a back specialist or as a neuromusculoskeletal specialist. Wardwell[21] maintains that chiropractic could, in fact, take one of five separate directions in the future:

1   It could fuse with medicine, either by joining it voluntarily (as did homeopathy and osteopathy) or by being taken over by medicine

2   It could be practised under medical supervision (as with physical therapists)

3   It could simply disappear

4   It could retain its present status as marginal or parallel to medicine

5   It could become a limited medical profession, such as dentistry, podiatry, and optometry.

For Wardwell, the fifth possibility reflects the reality of the way many chiropractors now practise and, furthermore, he sees this option as an attractive alternative, with advantages to the health-care system. In his opinion, chiropractic should compromise its original principles and become a limited medical profession. Within chiropractic itself, there is considerable support for Wardwell's conception of its future. Numerous writers have, in one form or another, postulated more constrained roles for chiropractic[27]. In many ways, the legitimacy of chiropractic has been achieved at the cost of a broader scope of chiropractic practice[28] and, by narrowing its scope of practice, chiropractic has gained greater legislative legitimacy.

The chiropractor as an alternate healer

At the same time that many chiropractors and social scientists are recommending a retrenchment of chiropractic, a new group of observers is also advancing its status as an alternative health-care paradigm and are exhorting the profession to protect and preserve that status[29,30].

Perhaps the fullest discussion of this issue, however, is given by Caplan[31]. His position is distinct in that his discussion begins with the premise that chiropractic is a unique and potentially valuable paradigm of health care. What others see as cultist, Caplan sees as a genuine alternative, intellectual paradigm: 'It seems that the chiropractic paradigm is not so much unscientific as it is a *different* science' [31]. Caplan's concern is that chiropractors are assisting in their own subjugation by giving up their unique paradigm. Unlike Wardwell, he sees strong social trends that will make this paradigm socially attractive. The self-care and holistic health-care movements are two trends that are contributing to the demand for alternative health care, and that embrace the ideas of chiropractic. Allied with this is the ongoing critique of medicine. With widespread popular support, he feels chiropractic has the opportunity to establish itself as equal to, but distinct from, traditional medicine.

Chiropractic health care

From the above literature, it is possible to draw some conclusions about chiropractic health care. Chiropractors have traditionally treated neuromusculoskeletal problems, but have expanded their care into what is now termed 'wellness' care. They have been involved with a variety of health problems, but these problems have seldom been the life-threatening, pathologic and traumatic conditions focused on by medicine. Even in the gastrointestinal and the viscerosomatic areas, chiropractors have focused on lifestyle-related problems (arising from stress, inappropriate diet, etc.). It may be argued, then, that chiropractors have been involved in wellness care as opposed to sick care. Few chiropractic patients die from the conditions presented to the chiropractor for treatment. From this perspective, the conflict between medicine and chiropractic (which at one level has been seen as the result of economic competition) has been misleading. Chiropractic has not competed successfully with medicine for illness care. The serious pathologies and traumas have always been treated predominantly by medicine and will, in all likelihood, continue to be so. Chiropractic has competed successfully in the area of functional pathology and lifestyle-related conditions (sprains and strains, posture, diet, exercise, etc.). Because this area is also of increased interest to health-care planners and the public, and because its focus would appear to be inherently preventive, chiropractic care offers an area for fruitful investigation. Chiropractic philosophy, with its concept of holistic care (mind, body, and spirit), would seem to give its clinical practice a decided edge over medicine in this regard.

How holistic is chiropractic?

Throughout this book we have stated that, at the level of philosophy, chiropractors endorse the concept of holism. In this chapter, we have noted that those researching the chiropractic health encounter have largely concurred with this assessment. It has become a *sine qua non* of the chiropractic profession that chiropractic, unlike medicine, treats the whole person. However, such a statement conceals more than it reveals. What is meant by the concept 'person' (or, even worse, the 'whole' person)? Are chiropractors capable of ever knowing the whole person? The latter involves two critical matters; one of philosophy (how can we know the other), and one of education (are chiropractors currently educated to enable them to know the other, and are they competent to do it in practice with regard to patients?). These are very complex questions. However, a genuine philosophy of chiropractic would challenge the blind acceptance by chiropractors of their most cherished belief, that they treat the whole person and not the disease[32].

To do this requires the examination of three fundamental concepts: the concept of holism, the concept of the person, and the concept of the individual. Part of the problem arises from the uncritical adoption of holism, at least philosophically, by the chiropractic profession.

The concept of holism

Holism accepts the uniqueness of each person. Allied with this belief is the assumption that the whole person, and the well person, involves the integration of the mind, body and spirit. Therefore, at the very least, it would require that the health provider is knowledgeable about biology, psychology, social science and spirituality, and have 'also experience, wisdom, compassion, and concern for the patient as a human being'[33]. Followed to its logical conclusion, such practice would involve the practitioner in the full range of social and cultural relationships of the patient, along with the complex spiritual dimensions of health. However, as Berliner and Salmon[34] note, if we examine the organizational structure of 'holistic' practice, we find that it also tends to be fee-for-service, entrepreneurial, serves largely a white middle-class population and has a sharp demarcation between the doctor and the patient. Holistic practitioners are just as likely to be as sexist and elitist as any other form of practitioner. Furthermore, while they may not focus on the disease and cells, they are reductionist in another sense in that they are almost entirely focused on the individual, with virtually no focus on the larger social groups. With regard to the concept of the person, this approach is reductionist. 'Persons' cannot be understood *qua* persons, apart from the social relationships they are a part of. To abstract persons out of these relationships is to reduce them as persons'[35].

One of the glaring deficiencies of holism is its failure to include such things as social classes and the political structure within its concept of illness, despite the clearly established influence of both on health. Holism cannot claim to consider the whole person, and then choose to leave out significant parts of the whole. A similar comment might also be made with respect to the treatment of the spiritual dimension, which would require a considerable knowledge of comparative religions to be practised successfully. Many holistic practitioners seem to assume that if they are spiritual, that solves the problem. Such an approach ignores the fact that it is the spirituality of the patient that is the concern, not that of the practitioner. In conclusion, while it is clear that holism does focus on the individual, it is less clear that this necessarily means holism focuses on the person or even less, the whole person.

The concept of the person

To understand this point, it is necessary to examine the concept of the person. First, it is necessary to recognize that patients viewed devoid of the social roles are denied the very thing that makes them individuals as opposed to biological beings. Humans are social beings; it is through social roles that they become part of the social fabric, and it is through roles that they develop an individual self and a personality[35]. While viewing the patient simply as a collection of body organs and processes misses the point of the individual, viewing the individual in isolation also misses the nature of personhood[36].

The concept of the individual

However, even viewing the patient in roles is insufficient to capture the full essence of the person. It is necessary to recognize that, over and above the roles we play, each person has both immutable rights and characteristics that are unique to them. This uniqueness can be described in numerous ways. Pellegrino[36] has argued that it lies in the possession of rationality – 'But to be an individual is not to be a person. It is in the possession of rationality as part of his nature that man becomes a person, an individual distinct from other individuals'[36]. Since rationality allows us to form our own ideas and judgements, it also allows us some freedom in choices. Because of this our choices will differ, and no two persons will make the exact same choices. 'Freedom is therefore the first obligation owed to persons *qua* persons'[36]. In this view, illness represents an assault on our ability to make free choices and, therefore, a fundamental assault on our 'person'. It is for this reason that illnesses with little pathology can be devastating in their impact on one patient, while patients with very serious pathology seem less affected. Pathology is a bad indicator of the impact of illness on the person, as opposed to its impact on the biology of the individual.

In illness, persons lack the knowledge and skill to help themselves and, therefore, must depend on others. Illness results in a diminution of the person and, in severe illness, may return the patient to an almost child-like dependency. Furthermore, it can be humiliating to the patient. In a very fundamental way, illness is an assault on the self and the self-image that the patient has constructed.

Knowing the patient

One solution to the problem of knowing the patient that has been adopted in medicine is to include the humanities in medical education. As Self[37] notes, there are two distinct pedagogical ways of doing this. In the first, the medical student is introduced to classical humanities with the hope that some enlightenment will rub off, and courses such as philosophy of medicine, history of medicine, literature and medicine, law and medicine, religion and medicine, and art and medicine would be included. In the second approach, formal courses are offered in humanistic psychology (stress management, interpersonal communication, professional burnout, introspection and self-concept development). Here, the emphasis is on developing sets of skills for the students to use in practice. The objective, therefore, is to produce physicians who will care for patients in a compassionate and humanistic manner, and this involves more than simply exposing the student to a little social science (such as psychology – the response used, for the most part, in chiropractic education). Such understanding is more likely to be found in the creative attempts of the artist to understand illness than in the writings of the scientists. In the case of the novelist, there is an attempt to know the other (and their illness) by an act of imaginative participation, and to share that experience with the reader. Great literature allows us to *live* the experience, and not simply to view it as an observer.

Chiropractic will therefore be humanistic and holistic only to the extent that the practitioner is able to understand the 'humanness' of the patient: 'One cannot expect doctors to attend to sick persons as persons, if they cannot describe them. Neither science nor medicine has the descriptive tools, but the humanities do'[38]. Disciplines like religion, philosophy and literature all deal with understanding the universal issues of life. For the doctor to help patients during the crisis of illness, some understanding of these issues is essential.

Although the humanities are a way of getting to know the 'other', and therefore the patient, they are not the only method. Within the social sciences there are paradigms that also allow us to do this, and these are often referred to as humanistic psychology or sociology, or interpretive sociology. For the most part, they have arisen from philosophical paradigms (e.g. phenomenology and American pragmaticism). They have also given rise to distinct methodological approaches (e.g. symbolic interactionism and ethnomethodology). These paradigms offer alternative investigative methods (qualitative methods)[39] that are more ideally suited to understanding and studying the patient, and these methods have been described elsewhere as 'holistic'[40]. The author has suggested in an earlier chapter that these paradigms provide an alternative to the empiricist approaches of the social sciences.

All of these areas of the humanities and the social sciences are notable for their absence in chiropractic education and, although some of the colleges have recently moved to requiring one prerequisite in both the humanities and the social sciences, this was not required historically. So unless we are to assume that chiropractors come by this skill of knowing the whole patient naturally, we should be somewhat sceptical as to the extent to which they are truly holistic.

From the above discussion it would seem that to know the patient involves considerably more than most chiropractors have been willing to admit. The profession cannot simply claim to treat the whole person without confronting the question of what that means. Furthermore, it must be able to demonstrate either that chiropractors are uniquely endowed with special empathetic skills, or that they are uniquely trained to achieve these. This should not be interpreted to mean that chiropractors have ignored the person. The philosophy of chiropractic has ensured that the worse reductionist excesses of biomedicine in ignoring the person have been avoided by chiropractic. However, all those alternative paradigms that claim to be holistic should be subjected to a critical philosophical examination of what such a claim means.

Conclusion

In evaluating the clinical role of the chiropractor, it is necessary to distinguish the context of the discussion. Much of the discussion in the literature to date has been about what chiropractors *might* become, *should* provide, or what *'chiropractic philosophy'* embraces, and have not been closely tied to empirical studies. Ultimately, the chiropractic role, and the clinical art of the chiropractor, are determined by what the patient brings to the chiropractor and what the patient will accept in terms of the treatment and care. No matter how holistic the chiropractor is, unless patients are willing to tolerate an intrusion into their private, social, and spiritual life, it is highly unlikely that chiropractors will be holistic practitioners. However, as the studies discussed in this chapter have shown, chiropractic patients have tolerated the establishment of wellness care around the limited health problems the patient actually brings to the practice, a broad-based wellness paradigm. As the above critique of the holistic claim makes clear, there are limitations to this holism, which should be acknowledged by both chiropractors and researchers. As discussed here, philosophy provides us a perspective for critically examining the holistic claim, not only of chiropractic but of all the alternative healers. What is clear from the discussion in this chapter is that portraying chiropractors simply as 'adjusters of backs' is a gross misunderstanding of the chiropractic paradigm.

References

[1] Hurwitz, E., Coulter, I. D., Adams, A. *et al.* (1998). Utilization of chiropractic care in the United States and Canada: 1985–1991. *Am. J. Publ. Health*, **88(5),** 771–6.

[2] Christensen, M. G. (ed.) (1993). *Job Analysis of Chiropractic. A Project Report, Survey Analysis and Summary of the Practice of Chiropractic within the United States.* National Board of Chiropractic Examiners.

[3] Shekelle, P. G., Markovich, M. and Louie, R. (1995). Comparing costs between provider types of episodes of back care pain. *Spine*, **20(2),** 221–7.

[4] Kelner, M., Hall, O. and Coulter, I. (1980). *Chiropractors: Do They Help?* Fitzhenry Whitesides.

[5] Coulehan, J. L. (1985). Chiropractic and the clinical art. *Soc. Sc. Med.*, **21(4),** 383–90.

[6] Jamison, J. R. (1993). Chiropractic holism: interactively becoming in a reductionist health care system. *Chiropr. J. Aust.*, **23(3),** 98–105.

[7] Jamison, J. R. (1997). An interactive model of chiropractic practice: reconstructing clinical reality. *J. Manipul. Physiol. Ther.*, **20(6),** 382–8.

[8] Jamison, J. R. (1997). Compliance or empowerment: an Australian case study. *Chiropr. J. Aust.*, **27(3),** 111–16.

[9] Coulter, I. D. (1990). The patient, the practitioner, and wellness: paradigm lost, paradigm gained. *J. Manipul. Physiol. Ther.*, **13(2),** 107–11.

[10] Coulter, I. D., Hays, R. D. and Danielson, C. D. (1996). The role of the chiropractor in the changing health-care system. From marginal to mainstream. *Res. Sociol. Health Care*, **13A,** 95–117.

[11] Coulter, I. D. (1996). Chiropractic approaches to wellness and healing. In *Advances in Chiropractic* (R. Mootz, ed.), pp. 431–46. Mosby.

[12] Gordon, J. S. (1980). The paradigm of holistic medicine. In *Health for the Whole Person* (A. C. Hastings, J. Fadiman and J. S. Gordon, eds), pp. 16–22. Westview Press.

[13] Coulter, I. D. (1993). A wellness system: the challenge for health professionals. *J. Can. Chiropr. Ass.*, **37(2),** 97–103.

[14] Seedhouse, D. (1986). *Health. The Foundations for Achievement.* John Wiley and Sons.

[15] Phillips, R. B., Coulter, I. D., Adams, A. *et al.* (1994). A contemporary philosophy of chiropractic for the Los Angeles College of Chiropractic. *J. Chiropr. Human.*, **4,** 20–25.

[16] Vernon, H. (1991). A model for incorporating the illness behavior model in the management of low back pain patients. *J. Manipul. Physiol. Ther.*, **14(6),** 379–89.

[17] Balduc, H. (1991). How chiropractic care can promote wellness. *Wellness Conference Northwestern College of Chiropractic.* Minneapolis St-Paul.

[18] Jamison, J. R. (1993). Acceptance and identity. The conundrum of contemporary chiropractic. *Chiropr. J. Aust.*, **23,** 136–40.

[19] Jamison, J. R. (1991). *Health Promotion for Chiropractic Practice*. Aspen Publishers.

[20] Kranz, C. K. (1995). An overview of primary care concepts. *Topics Clin. Chiropr.*, **21**, 55–65.

[21] Wardwell, W. (1980). The present and future role of chiropractic. In *Modern Developments in the Principles and Practice of Chiropractic* (S. Haldeman, ed.), pp. 25–41. Appleton-Century-Croft.

[22] Coulter, I. D. (1992). Is chiropractic care primary health care? *J. Can. Chiropr. Ass.*, **36(2)**, 96–101.

[23] Callahan, D. and Cianciulli, A. (1994). *The Chiropractor as a Primary Health Care Provider in Rural, Health Professional Shortage Areas of the US*. FCER Publication Number 9452, Foundation for Chiropractic Education and Research.

[24] Bowers, L. J. and Mootz, R. D. (1995). The nature of primary care: the chiropractors role. *Topics Clin. Chiropr.*, **2(1)**, 66–84.

[25] Council on Chiropractic Education (1987). *Educational Standards for Chiropractic Colleges*. Council on Chiropractic Education.

[26] Haldeman, S., Chapman-Smith, D. and Petersen, D. (1992). *Guidelines for Chiropractic Quality Assurance and Practice Parameters*. Aspen Publishers.

[27] DeBoer, K. and Waagen, G. (1986). The future role of the chiropractor in the health-care system. *J. Manipul. Physiol. Ther.*, **9**, 225–8.

[28] Coburn, D. (1991). Legitimacy at the expense of narrowing of scope of practice in Canada. *J. Manipul. Physiol. Ther.*, **14(10)**, 14–21.

[29] Evans, G. D. (1973). A sociology of chiropractic. *J. Can. Chiropr. Ass.*, **21**, 6–18.

[30] Morinis, F. A. (1980). Theory and practice of chiropractic: an anthropological perspective. *J. Can. Chiropr. Ass.*, **24**, 114–19.

[31] Caplan, R. L. (1984). Chiropractic. In *Alternative Medicine: Popular and Policy Perspectives* (J. Salmon, ed.), pp. 86–7. Tavistock.

[32] Coulter, I. D. (1993). The physician, the patient, and the person: the humanistic challenge. *J. Chiropr. Human.*, **1**, 9–20.

[33] Gordon, J. S. (1980). The paradigm of holistic medicine. In *Health for the Whole Person* (A. C. Hastings, J. Fadiman and J. S. Gordon, eds), pp. 16–22. Westview Press.

[34] Berliner, H. S. and Salmon, J. W. (1980). The holistic alternative to scientific medicine: history and analysis. *Int. J. Health Serv.*, **1**, 133–47.

[35] MacIntyre, A. (1979). Medicine aimed at the care of persons rather than what . . .? In *Changing Values in Medicine* (E. J. Cassell and M. Siegler, eds), pp. 93–98. University Publishers of America.

[36] Pellegrino, E. D. (1979). Philosophical groundings for treating the patient as a person: a commentary on Alisdair MacIntyre. In *Changing Values in Medicine* (E. J. Cassell and M. Siegler, eds), pp. 99–103. University Publishers of America.

[37] Self , D. (1988). The pedagogy of two different approaches to humanistic medical education: cognitive vs. affective. *Theor. Med.*, **9**, 227–36.

[38] Weston, W. W. (1988). The person: a missing dimension in medical care and medical education. *Can. Fam. Phys.*, **34**, 1701–1803.

[39] Mealing, D. (1998). Quantitative, qualitative and emergent approaches to chiropractic research: a philosophical background. *J. Manipul. Physiol. Ther.*, **21(3)**, 205–11.

[40] Coulter, I. D., Adams, A., Coogan, P. *et al.* (1998). A comparative study of chiropractic and medical education. *Alt. Ther. Health Med.*, **4(5)**, 64–75.

CHAPTER 6

Chiropractic and medicine as distinct health encounters

In examining the future of chiropractic, it is instructive to consider the past. So much of chiropractic history and the philosophy of chiropractic developed as a response to medicine that it is essential to understand how these two paradigms have evolved over the past 100 years. Furthermore, it is in the differences between these two paradigms that we can begin to understand why chiropractic, and alternative health care, has not only survived but is flourishing in modern society. It is also here that we may begin to understand what the future holds for chiropractic.

Medicine in the twentieth century

The roots of the great success of medicine in this century are to be found in the nineteenth century, in the emergence of the germ theory of disease[1]. The theory brought science and medicine into a partnership that was to transform the nature of medicine. The spectacular results that were obtained from the application of the theory in the search for the causes of disease provided the foundation for the dominance of the medical paradigm in western society. It gave, for the first time, the possibility of therapeutically impacting on the killer diseases. However, more importantly, it gave a new methodology – that of science – for approaching disease. Increasingly, medicine became less a purely clinical matter and more a matter of science and therapy, and the search for wonder drugs. The successful attack on bacilli and viruses was dependent on the development of pharmacology, and antibiotics and inoculation gave medicine some spectacular achievements in the age-old fight against disease. As well as developments in surgery and technology, medicine began to confront the problem of degeneration. The most dramatic change has occurred with regard to organ transplants, but techniques of surgical removal and repair were just as important.

The historical trend, therefore, was from the clinical art of medicine to the science of medicine, a change reflected also in the name of medical faculties and buildings. In most universities, the buildings are now called the 'medical sciences' building.

Along with its successes, however, medicine also paid a price. The successes were increasingly with acute illnesses and trauma, as opposed to chronic illness. More and more, its therapies involved radical forms of interventions, which had associated iatrogenic costs. The more radical the therapy, the higher the risks arising from it and the more likely there are to be drastic side effects (as in chemotherapy, for example). Furthermore, as science came to play a significant role in medicine, so too did medicine become increasingly dependent on basic and applied scientific research and technology. A result of the latter is that the site for medical practice changed, and the hospitals that were once simply nursing institutions controlled by nurses became the power houses of the new medicine controlled, until very recently, by medical doctors. This century marked the decline in importance of the solo medical practitioner, and the home visit virtually ceased to exist. The solo practice has become the group practice and, increasingly, resembles a hospital clinic in technology.

As for patients, the achievements in health gains and longevity have been considerable. However, the gains have not been without some costs. As the focus moved to germs and the biological structures of the body, two things occurred: first, the focus on the patient as a person was lost, and second, whole areas of concern to health, particularly social and cultural factors, were excluded. What was not reducible to biology became of less priority. The very success of the germ theory of disease introduced limitations to the medical paradigm.

Along with the reductionism inherent in this biologically based paradigm came specialization among the providers. The area of diagnosis expanded, and increasingly moved out of the hands of the medical provider as both technology and other professions came to be inserted into the health encounter. The focus on so-called 'killer diseases' also meant a focus on what are frequently irreversible pathologies. The very successes of the paradigm also highlight the failures, as in the case of the war on cancer. Such diseases have not succumbed to the methods of the paradigm in the way that, for example, infectious diseases did. The failures are also made more problematic because the successes. Wonder drugs and technology lead to the expectation for miracles and cures, and the expectations of patients have been elevated by the very successes of the paradigm. When this is combined with the critiques of medicine discussed earlier, medicine finds itself in the peculiar position at the end of the twentieth century of being more successful in treating disease than it has ever been, while at the same time being more extensively criticized and experiencing the steady erosion of its influence. Medicine finds itself being attacked despite its great achievements and, in some ways, because of them.

The important factor in this history is not the germ theory of disease as such, but the orientation to disease and treatment (the paradigm) that was ushered in with the theory. This orientation had vast social ramifications. It not only transformed the social settings of medicine, but it fundamentally altered the doctor–patient relationship. While the treatment procedures have been increasingly rationalized, this has been done at the cost of human relationships. Hospitals may deliver highly scientific and rationalized medicine, but they are often very alienating social structures for patients. Radical therapy may save lives, but it may also have debilitating side effects for the patient. Therefore, what at first appeared a simple change in the theoretical basis of medicine had vast ramifications for the whole system of health care.

Medical education

Educationally, medicine moved from proprietary institutions into universities. In North America, this came about through the influence of the 1910 *Flexner Report*, which not only resulted in the closing of many of the medical schools but also helped to locate medicine in the university. Increasingly, medicine became dependent on two institutions – the university and the teaching hospital. The latter became a two-way dependency, with the university depending on the hospital for clinical education and the hospital dependent on the medical school for students and residents as a source of staffing.

The location of education in these two institutions had numerous consequences for medicine. Both are costly institutions, and require huge amounts of money to operate. In modern universities, the budget of the medical school will generally be greater than that of any other faculty by several magnitudes. However, the university is not controlled by the medical profession, and therefore the educational programme can develop in ways that may not be the most appropriate for a medical practitioner, particularly for general practice. In the past 20 years this has been seen in the great shortage of primary care doctors in America, which has resulted from medical schools focusing on specialists. University curricula and university departments have their own growth dynamics, and the tendency is to expand rather than to contract. Medical education has become lengthy and costly. By tying medicine to science, medical education has been impacted by the knowledge explosion that has occurred in this century in the sciences. Increasingly, a medical school curriculum has come to include a vast amount of basic and biological science, whatever its relevance to actual practice. The increasing dependence of medicine on scientifically generated therapies is reflected in the role of science in the curriculum. Not only do medical students have to master large amounts of science during their training; increasingly, a premed education is also in the sciences. Medicine has come to recruit science-oriented students for a person-oriented profession.

Neither the university nor the teaching hospital provides the typical setting that many doctors will practice in, the general practice. Compared to general practice, the general hospital is an exotic location. It contains a range of expensive and elaborate technology, much of which is not available in general practice. This also increasingly tied the general practitioner to the specialists and hospitals, to obtain the services for their patients.

Both universities and teaching hospitals tend to be large and impersonal social organizations. Within the universities, the popularity of medicine (and the resources it was able to garner from the state) means that the size of the medical faculty is limited only by the restrictions placed on enrolment numbers, and even then, only a fraction of applicants succeed in finding a place. In some schools, only 1 in 10 of all applicants make it into medical school. It is instructive that in the US, despite what is seen as an over supply of physicians, no medical schools have been closed. This is in stark contrast to dentistry where, through actual closures and enrolment reductions, the equivalent of 20 schools of dentistry have been closed in the US in the past 10 years. Because of this, academic excellence, both before admission and during the first years of medical school, has become the dominant factor in the selection of future medical physicians. However, this leads to a conflict between the two settings. In the university, the excellence refers to academic excellence and is measured by the ability to master the knowledge of the sciences. In the hospital, excellence refers to clinical performance, and there may not necessarily be any relationship between this and academic performance.

The scientific orientation of twentieth century medicine has also resulted in the development of its research paradigm. In both the university and the hospital there have developed the research programmes that have come to characterize modern medicine. The funding for this research has also become the engine driving the development of medical education since, over time, the externally funded research has come to greatly outstrip the educational budget of medical schools. Tuition represents a very small contribution to the overall income of a medical school. Research-generated knowledge, particularly in the form of random controlled trials, has come to represent the gold standard in modern medicine. In contemporary terminology, evidence-based practice is the goal of medicine. The fact that the clinical challenges always greatly outstrip the amount of evidence seems often to be overlooked. However, with the great explosion in knowledge, the need to specialize has also grown. As twentieth century medicine has expanded, so too has the number of specialists. This provides the medical student with a wide variety of career paths other than general practice. Furthermore, the status of the specialist in the university and teaching hospital has come to far exceed that of the general practitioner, making it increasingly likely that students will choose a specialty rather than general practice on graduation.

The teaching hospital

The teaching hospital is not only an exotic setting; it also tends to be a tertiary hospital whose focus is on acute illness and trauma. This has had at least two consequences for medical education. First, it has led to an overwhelming concentration on illnesses and trauma that do not form the bulk of general practice. The student trains on sick people who are at the point of needing the services of the hospital – the very point at which the services of a general practitioner have been superseded. Second, the students are involved in the more negative consequences of illness, death and debilitation. In many ways, modern hospitals have become the institutions where people die, but only after heroic efforts to save them. In such a situation, it is imperative that medical novices develop a form of detachment and clinical objectivity that protects them from being overwhelmed with grief. Added to this is the realization that mistakes by them while using radical therapies can hasten death. In this setting, patients have increasingly come to be seen as cases or, even worse, as interesting teaching cases rather than as persons. Mr Smith has become 'the bypass in Ward 2'. In the hospital setting, a case has a peculiar connotation. A case here is an exemplar of a particular disease or traumatic injury and, on this basis, interns and residents look forward to experiencing interesting, exciting cases.

There have been other consequences of locating the internship and residencies of medical students in the teaching hospitals. Hospitals by their nature stress interdisciplinary treatment, and a whole host of functionaries are able to assist in conducting tests, therapies etc. While this may result in effective care, it means that numerous functionaries intervene between the doctor and the patient, reducing both the intimacy of the doctor–patient relationship and the comprehensiveness of the relationship. When tasks are delegated, so, too, are parts of the relationship.

Hospital care also constitutes a very concentrated part of a person's illness. There is usually a history of illness and care prior to hospital admittance and a history afterwards and, for the most part, the medical intern will experience neither. Interns/residents may play no part in the initial acceptance of the patient or in the initial determination of a person as a patient, a significant part of illness as opposed to disease. They may also play no part in managing the patient after discharge from the hospital. Even in the hospital, the intern will not manage the care. By their nature, teaching hospitals are not in the business of holistic care and, despite the number of deaths that occur in tertiary hospitals, they are also not really in the business of managing death. This fact has given rise to the development of hospices. When the tertiary hospital has completed its task (and success is measured partly by discharge), the patient is usually returned to some other provider (generally to whoever referred them). In the case of specialists, the care may continue past discharge, but is expected to terminate when the particular health problem has been resolved. The expectation is not of a long-term relationship with the patient. Termination in the hospital is likely to be fairly abrupt; the patient can either die or get discharged. In many cases the termination occurs once the hospital has established the actual diagnosis, or it occurs immediately the patient can cope without the elaborate facilities of the hospital. This may be a considerable time before the illness has been terminated. Under the new forms of managed care, this period has been drastically reduced for all illnesses in hospitals. A case in the hospital, from this perspective, is a very truncated affair.

As noted above, a key role of the modern hospital (and a key feature of modern medicine) is accurate diagnosis. This is achieved in contemporary medicine through the use of complex and sophisticated technology. However, once the diagnosis has been obtained, the treatment may be quite standardized. Once the physician knows the patient has diabetes, and how serious it is, there are acceptable standards of care that the provider is expected to follow (and they can be sued if they do not). Furthermore, much of the therapy is carried out by others, not the physician. For the most part, tertiary hospitals are for problems that admit speedy solutions rather than for long-term, chronic problems. These are handled in other institutions which, although the medical student may be exposed to them, will not constitute a significant part of their education.

Summary

In summary, the marriage of medicine to the university and the associated teaching hospital, while it conferred significant advantages, did not come without its costs. The main advantage is that it introduced a science-based education, which not only improved the practice of medicine but also conferred significant prestige and political power on the profession. Furthermore it introduced a common clinical education, which has gone a long way to ensuring both the quality of medical education post-Flexner and also the quality of medical practice, by ensuring a minimum set of clinical skills a physician should possess. However, it is an education that, until very recently, has focused on understanding and treating disease and trauma rather than on the management of health. Health in this paradigm became the absence of disease. Again until very recently, medical education did not seem to be ideally suited to the notion of general practice, and in fact general practice (in terms of status in the university) was seen as somewhere at the bottom of the totem pole. It is important to note that medicine itself is currently responding vigorously to these issues. Specialties in general practice and family medicine have emerged, medical schools now own and participate in community practices and clinics, some medical schools have returned their mission to the graduation of general practitioners, and new groups in holistic medicine and integrative medicine have emerged within the profession. However, these are developments of the last part of the twentieth century, and do not fundamentally challenge the history outlined above.

One consequence of the relationship between the university and the hospital is that medical students are provided with a large captive pool of patients on which to learn. They do not face the problems of recruiting and retaining patients as clients – a fairly important skill for a doctor to survive in private practice. The development of important interpersonal skills was not an essential component for survival.

Chiropractic in the twentieth century

Chiropractic followed a quite different route of development to that of medicine. First, its focus was not on disease, serious pathology or trauma. Chiropractic concerned itself with functional problems, largely of neuromusculoskeletal origin. These health problems were often biomechanical, but with neurological impacts. Even where chiropractic focused on visceral somatic problems, it was ones that could be related, at least theoretically, to neural problems caused by spinal impingement. Chronic problems were a significant part of the chiropractic focus. To a large extent, the acute problems that chiropractors dealt with (such as back pain) are reversible and in fact have a natural history of righting themselves if left alone. Although chiropractors developed a range of adjunctive therapies, one group (the straights) confined themselves to manipulation of the spine only with the hand only. Furthermore, for the most part the adjunctive therapies were secondary to adjustments, and were frequently used as a way of preparing the patient for adjustment. Chiropractic remains overwhelmingly a manual therapy. Chiropractors also remain drugless and non-surgical. The former is complicated somewhat by the widespread use of supplements and natural herbs by chiropractors, but all these are non-prescriptive drugs. The fact that they have remained drugless and non-surgical may be as much a matter of opportunity as commitment, although many of the profession remain adamantly opposed to prescribing drugs. By being excluded from universities and hospitals by the lobbying of medicine, surgery was never a political option for chiropractic, irrespective of what the profession may have thought about it.

Science and chiropractic

As noted earlier in the book, the relationship between science and chiropractic was also fundamentally different to that in medicine. Initially, in both medicine and chiropractic, science played a legitimizing role. Both types of providers were educated in science, not because the practices of either were particularly scientific, but because scientific education was used to cloak both in the mantle of respectability. Over time, however, science began to play a much more central role in medicine in that it became the basis of the research paradigm. In many ways, the great achievements of medicine in this century have come out of this research arm. This does not imply that all modern medicine is scientifically based; it is clearly not, and some estimate that only about 10 per cent of medical procedures have any scientific basis. However, few (if any) chiropractic therapies were derived from scientific research; they were empirically based, just as they had been for most of medicine's history. Science was used in chiropractic *post hoc* to provide support for the theoretical concepts, and the major therapies in chiropractic did not arise out of scientific research. This contrasts vividly to drug therapy and areas such as kidney transplants, where basic science has played a crucial role. This can be seen in such areas as the resolving of tissue rejection in organ transplants. Chiropractic therefore did not develop the dependency that medicine has on science in the twentieth century. The development of its therapies has remained firmly in the hands of chiropractors. One of the reasons for this is there is in a sense no science of the spine. The sciences of anatomy, physiology, neurology, biomechanics and kinesiology all contribute to our understanding of the spine, but they do not generate therapies in the way that, for example, drug research does. These sciences enter chiropractic in the form of theories to provide rationale for therapies, but they did not originally create the therapies themselves. In the case of manipulation, the therapies have been developed overwhelmingly by practitioners. It is here that chiropractors have been at their most creative. Unlike medicine, where diagnoses have been the climactic events of this century, in chiropractic it has been the elaboration of therapy. The basis of this development has not been science, but rather what works (practice empiricism). To remove the science-generated therapies from modern medicine would be to destroy much of its therapeutic power, whereas to remove them in chiroprac-tic would have little impact on the practice in the area of manipulation. With regard to nutrition, stress management, exercise, etc., chiropractors draw on the same science as medicine and other health providers. As a corollary of this lack of dependence on science, chiropractic also did not develop the technical jargon of science. Chiropractors' explanations tend to be metaphor-based and compre-hensible to their patients, and they tend to use simple anatomical models, charts or X-rays. While it did develop its own language and concepts (e.g. subluxation), these seem to be more accessible to patients and friendlier than the terminology of science and medicine. While this relationship to science has had negative consequences for chiropractic, it has also had a tremendous positive effect. It is due to the rush to science that medicine became highly reductionistic, non-holistic, used radical interventions and lost much of its humanism. Many of the ills of modern medicine have arisen from its wholesale embrace of science.

Chiropractic focus

Because the focus has not been on disordered pathology but on 'functional pathology', chiropractors have been concerned with the total functioning of the body as an integral unit and with threats to the integrity of that unit. Their paradigm orientates them in this direction. These threats or insults to the functioning of the body are to be found and corrected in the lifestyle of the patient. They may arise from accidents, but may equally be due to poor posture, sleeping habits, diet and lack of or inappropriate exercise. These insults can be identified and corrected in large part by the patient. The chiropractor provides the manipulation that gives short-term relief of pain, but the patient must participate in long-term correction of the behaviour causing the problem. In a sense, the chiropractor has a double advantage here. First, much of what they deal with is reversible, and often within a short time. However, they are also able to intervene at the level of lifestyle both to correct the problem and prevent future occurrences. These are often simple interventions that patients can accomplish readily (such as not sleeping on their stomach, changing their work chair, removing bulky wallets from their hip pocket, etc.). So the visit involves both health treatment (manipulation) and also health care (lifestyle intervention) that will occur outside the visit and without the practitioner, thus reinforcing the concept of holistic care. This is something much more difficult to achieve when one is dealing with serious pathology or trauma, even if the providers' paradigm was oriented in this manner.

Although chiropractic could have focused on all types of ailments, given its philosophy of health, in fact it has focused on a very narrow range. Overwhelmingly, these have been problems associated with the spine. Although the initial theories of chiropractic postulated that these problems were implicated in many forms of illness, the outstanding feature of chiropractic in the twentieth century is that it came to focus on spinal problems as problems in their own right. At the theoretical level, the bodies of knowledge on which chiropractors have drawn extensively are anatomy, neurology, physiology, bio-mechanics and kinesiology.

One outstanding result of the chiropractic focus on the spine is that chiropractors can obtain results with their therapy that are usually readily apparent to their patients. This is quite different from having to deal with irreversible pathologies. Although chiropractors are exposed to the full range of illnesses in their patients, they are not primarily responsible for treating most of them. Death and debilitating illness does not often intrude into a chiropractic office. A consequence of this is that the chiropractic paradigm is able to embrace a very positive notion of the body's ability to heal; something difficult to achieve in the case of the terminally ill. At their level of work, chiropractors are able to experience the reinforcement that comes from seeing the body restore itself without the aid of radical intervention. In the case of chronic illness, they are able to experience partnership with patients over the long term, helping the patients to cope with and manage their disabilities. Chiropractic practice, therefore, as a result of the historical focus, provides strong reinforcement for the chiropractic philosophy of health and health care. In many ways it acts as a self-fulfilling prophecy for the practitioner, and is reflected in the different level of confidence that chiropractors express in their ability to assist with back pain when compared to that of doctors[2].

Another major characteristic of chiropractic in the twentieth century is that it did not become hospital based. This is partly due to the fact that chiropractors do not treat serious acute illness or trauma, but it is also a result of being excluded by medicine. Chiropractic care, unlike medicine, has remained in solo practices or small joint practices, and has not developed the more alienating structures of the large hospitals. Furthermore, in chiropractic few intermediaries intervene between the chiropractor and the patient. This is not a practice where the patient is referred to the pharmacist for the treatment. Chiropractic care overwhelmingly involves the chiropractor doing something to the patient on each visit, usually through personal touch[3].

Diagnosis

Unlike medicine, the elaborate, highly technical system of diagnosis did not emerge in chiropractic. While the chiropractor may use X-rays and laboratory tests, the essential diagnosis is a physical one. In this regard, chiropractic, with its emphasis on palpatory skills and physical observation, resembles medical practice in the days of home visits – the physician with a little black bag. In the days when physicians made home visits, they were highly dependent on their own ability to conduct a physical diagnosis. In a very similar way, chiropractic has had to evolve a form of practice where diagnosis does not usually involve a wide range of complicated tests carried out by machines or other health providers. This is partly a reflection of choice made by chiropractic, but also reflects the fact that, in neuromusculoskeletal health problems, definitive diagnosis is neither available nor currently possible.

Side effects

Owing to the nature of chiropractic therapy, and the fact that it is conservative, it seldom has radical side effects. The risk from manipulation is calculated at 4.6 serious complications per 1 000 000 adjustments. This compares to 6 deaths per 1000 back operations[4]. Because it deals with conditions that are reversible, many of which also will recover spontaneously, chiropractic tends to get good results for the patient.

Chiropractic education

Chiropractic education, like the practice, has followed a different route from that of medicine[5]. The contrast in the settings for education for the two professions could hardly be greater. Where medicine became fixed in the university setting, chiropractic (until very recently, and then only in a small group of colleges) was systematically excluded from universities largely because of medical opposition. In addition, chiropractic, for virtually all of its history, has received no state funding. Chiropractic colleges began as proprietary institutions surviving on student tuition fees. Although they are now non-proprietary, they are still overwhelmingly private, non-profit-making institutions, dependent on student tuition for funding. This isolation from university settings has impacted on chiropractic in many ways, but one major impact is that it has never enjoyed the vast intellectual resources that have been put at the disposal of medicine and that are not part of the medical profession as such. Chiropractic educational institutions have remained modest in terms of facilities, nowhere near approaching those of medical schools. Their facilities are less costly than medicine and, in areas such as laboratories and libraries, are clearly inferior. As a consequence, of course, it costs a lot less to educate a chiropractor. Furthermore, chiropractic colleges are not associated with teaching hospitals. When compared to medicine, chiropractic would seem greatly disadvantaged. However, facilities do not by themselves determine the quality of a programme or of the graduates. If they did, the students who studied under the ancient Greek philosophers would also have been disadvantaged.

While the isolation from university has had costs for chiropractic, in other ways it has conferred some advantages.

As the profession in a sense owns the educational institutions, it has been able to exercise direct control over the content of the education. This has meant that, in chiropractic, the education programme has remained much more closely tied to the needs of the practitioner. The profession has been able to influence directly the elaboration of the various types of knowledge and, unlike universities, where esoteric bodies of knowledge can be expanded without any relationship to their pragmatic usefulness, the chiropractic colleges have remained much more geared to the graduation of general practitioners. Within chiropractic colleges, what has developed is the types of knowledge relevant to chiropractic. The basic sciences in chiropractic have functioned in a service capacity and have nowhere been permitted to develop in ways determined by the particular discipline. A physiologist teaching in a chiropractic college would seldom, if ever, be developing a major research programme for the advancement of physiology. In the university setting, departments and disciplines have their own growth dynamics that may or may not have relevance for the practice of medicine. The notion of developing knowledge for its own sake, so-called 'pure science', is a luxury chiropractic colleges have not been able to afford. In universities, not only is such knowledge pursued, but it also tends to expand so that, over time, the demands made for areas of content come to overwhelm the curriculum. While on the one hand chiropractic research has been meagre and is still modest, and funding very limited, on the other, chiropractic colleges have not been burdened with the costs of elaborate but expensive research facilities. Furthermore, they do not constantly lose some of their brightest students to research.

Partly as a reflection of the reality of chiropractic practice, and its exclusion from hospitals, the great drive towards producing specialists did not occur in chiropractic colleges. They remain, even after a 100-year history, institutions for educating general practitioners. Even where they offer post-graduate specialties, such as roentgenology, they offer only one or two residency-based programmes. The rest are offered as continuing education programmes, carried out by persons in practice. Frequently those who take such courses continue work in general practice, although they have advanced education in certain areas. Chiropractic is in the peculiar situation that, while it does produce specialists, it does not produce specialties in the sense that medicine does. The profession has not become fragmented amongst the specialties in the way medicine has, and the dominant political force in the profession is still the rank-and-file generalists.

The chiropractic clinic

Where medicine developed the teaching hospital as the major clinical site for education, chiropractic colleges developed an out-patient, ambulatory clinic. These clinics were set up and organized along the lines of a general practice, with largely the same equipment. Chiropractic students train in settings very similar to those in which they will practise, and they also gain experience in the ways they will practise. The chiropractic teaching clinic is different from the methods used in medicine in another sense. Here, the student is responsible for recruiting many of the patients. Because of the historical position of chiropractic, very few (if any) colleges were able to adopt a policy of 'build it and they will come', and even today few of the colleges could guarantee sufficient walk-in patients for the students to complete their clinical education. The students therefore learn another essential skill for graduation; building up a patient clientele. Furthermore, since these teaching clinics are mostly on college grounds and are all owned and operated by the colleges even when off the campus, there is no contradiction between the learning experience in the college and the clinical experience. This does not imply perfect harmony between the two. It is still possible for the student to learn practices in the teaching clinic that they have been taught in the didactic programme have no validity, but the differences between the two are insignificant compared to those in medicine. One of the downsides of the students recruiting the patients is that the patient population can be atypical of real practice. Students tend to recruit friends or acquaintances, the majority of whom are young and relatively healthy.

The experience in the clinic is also distinct. In a chiropractic clinic, the patients are seldom acutely ill or have serious pathology or trauma. They are ambulatory and, for the most part, have not been referred there. This means that being accepted in the patient role begins in the teaching clinic, which, although true in the emergency and outpatient departments, is not true for most patients admitted to hospital. Similarly, the termination of the case is likely to be in the chiropractic clinic. Chiropractic students therefore do not have a truncated case, but get to manage the whole case – they have the totality of the illness episode available to them. Furthermore, in chiropractic colleges the student manages the case (although under supervision) and, to a degree not true of medical students (even in their residencies), the patient belongs to the chiropractic student. The student is able to develop a relationship with patients as their primary provider in the clinic. This management occurs with the type of patients and problems that will make up the bulk of practice. The weakness is that such clinics (and therefore the student) will not be exposed to serious pathology and disease, which on occasion also turns up in a chiropractic office. The clinical education of the chiropractor is therefore almost the reverse of that of a medical doctor. The latter train on the seriously ill who, for the most part, constitute a small part of a general practice (but not of course of hospital or specialty practice). Chiropractors are trained on the less ill, who constitute the bulk of general practice, but they do not learn how to manage the seriously ill. One consequence of this is that the students do not develop the types of psychological defence mechanisms, the clinical detachment, learned by most medical students.

As a consequence of the clinical setting, the chiropractic student is involved in all aspects of the doctor–patient relationship. This is reinforced by the fact that the student must also recruit and retain patients. In this model, students have to pay attention to the needs of the patient since, in a sense, the power lies with the patient. If the patient leaves, the student fails to complete the required number of patients and/or procedures required for graduation.

Last but not least, although the teaching clinic may be large the student acts largely as a 'solo' practitioner. The student conducts the history taking and makes the diagnosis, determines the tests required, carries out the therapy and determines the termination. While all of this is of course under supervision, the essential feature is that the student is the 'doctor' and where others intrude it is in a supervisory capacity and rarely at the therapeutic level. While the student may request help from a supervising clinician at any stage, the overwhelming pattern is for the student to conduct the care.

Summary

In examining the content of the education, while the courses taught in both chiropractic and medicine appear very similar, particularly with regard to science, there is a major difference in the relationship of science to therapies. As noted earlier, chiropractic students must take science prerequisites before entrance into a Chiropractic College, and the first 2 years of the programme are overwhelmingly concerned with the basic and biological sciences. In chiropractic, the sciences provide the rationales for practice. There is therefore a very pragmatic orientation to the sciences. Those areas of most relevance – such as neurology, physiology and anatomy – form a core part of the programme. However, the sciences are not taught here as the source of therapies. Science may explain the therapies and their impact, but seldom have therapies in chiropractic been developed as the result of research in the basic and biological sciences. In a sense, this is *post hoc* science. Historically, the therapies came first and the science followed.

In conclusion, therefore, what appeared at first to be serious disadvantages for chiropractic education were in some ways blessings in disguise. It is clear that chiropractors have been able to develop educational institutions that produce graduates who obtain high levels of state and public acceptability and patient loyalty. This implies that chiropractors were able to overcome the severe limitations they experienced in terms of resources.

The chiropractic and medical health encounter

It is at the level of the patient health encounter that we need to examine what difference any of this has made. Our earlier chapter examined the features of the chiropractic health encounter; this section will continue that exploration, but counterpoises the chiropractic encounter with the medical one. The method used here is termed by sociologist 'ideal types'. That is, while it recognizes that all health encounters will vary, the method attempts to abstract the essential features of most encounters. No encounter will be exactly what is described here, but all will resemble it in some way.

In the study by Kelner and colleagues[5], numerous methods were used to collect the data on the health encounter. They included administering questionnaires to both patients and chiropractors, observing the treatment of patients, detailed vignettes of selected patients, and placing a researcher as a participant observer in a treatment programme over a 1-year period. From all this data, the authors constructed a model of the encounter that involves seven distinct stages. While all encounters will vary in some ways, the purpose of such a model is to extract the dominant features with enough generality that both the patients and the chiropractors identify them as general features of the encounter. They are intended to capture the essence of the encounter in chiropractic, not the exact encounter of all patients. It is in this sense that the model is considered an ideal type. The seven stages are as follows:

1   The initial contact

2   The formulation of a diagnosis

3   The chiropractor's explanation to the patient

4   The negotiation of a treatment plan

5   The delivery of care (treatment)

6   Evaluation of the effects of treatment

7   Termination of the case.

We will compare and contrast these seven stages in chiropractic and medicine.

The initial contact

In medicine the initial visit is conventional in that, in our culture, this is an interaction that is highly structured and is known to the participants. Even if the person has never visited this particular medical physician (or any medical physician), the encounter is portrayed extensively on our television and in movies, literature etc. Medical practice is deeply embedded in our culture, and most of us know what to expect, and what is acceptable and unacceptable behaviour by the physician. Most people have a medical doctor and will have had one from birth, or at least visited one since. A lifetime of socialization has educated us as to what a medical doctor does, what problems we should take there, and what is likely in broad terms to happen while we are there.

In contrast, when making the first contact with the chiropractor, individuals must make the decision to step outside mainstream health care and to select a form of health care that has historically been described in very unflattering terms by medical physicians. Chiropractors are seldom portrayed in our media and, for most individuals, the first visit may be the very first exposure to chiropractic. The first visit is therefore problematic in a way that the visit to the medical physician is not. For example, such questions as whether or not patients disrobe in a chiropractic office, what kind of examination will be performed, what a chiropractic office looks like and what the chiropractic will actually do are all unanswered prior to the visit. For the chiropractor the initial visit is crucial, because there is not only the challenge of diagnosing the problem and deciding if it can be treated, but also of introducing the patient to chiropractic itself. This first visit may not only decide if the person becomes a patient, but whether he or she will become the patient of any chiropractor. A medical physician may have to convince patients about their problem and its seriousness (or lack of seriousness) but, for the most part, does not have to convince them about the legitimacy of medicine. The medical doctor can focus on convincing the person about the legitimacy of the treatment. For new patients, the chiropractic encounter often starts at a step prior to that; establishing the legitimacy of chiropractic itself.

Contributing to this is the fact that a large percentage of chiropractic patients (research shows that this ranges from 30–60 per cent) have tried some other form of health care for the particular problem prior to coming to chiropractic. This is overwhelmingly mainstream care, predominantly medical. Failing to get results, patients come to the chiropractor seeking an alternative solution. In many cases, they may also feel rejected as malingerers or as having psychosomatic illness when no cause could be found. For these patients, the first visit may be the first time their status as a 'patient' is conferred, a status that legitimizes their illness.

In the chiropractic first visit there is therefore a considerable 'sizing up' being carried out by both the patient and the provider. Not only are they evaluating one another as people; the chiropractor is trying to determine if this is a patient who is manageable or hostile, resistant or co-operative, as well as determining whether the problem is treatable by chiropractic. In chiropractic, the first visit tends to be lengthy.

The diagnosis

The procedures at the first visit may be simple or elaborate but, even at its most elaborate, the process of deriving a diagnosis in chiropractic is distinct from that of medicine. A chiropractic diagnosis tends to be tentative, is based on observation rather than definitive tests, is narrower in focus and is carried out almost entirely by the chiropractor. This partly reflects the fact that in neuromusculoskeletal problems (unlike, for example, diabetes), a definitive diagnosis is not possible. While the chiropractor may use X-rays or laboratory tests to rule out pathology, overwhelmingly the chiropractic diagnosis is derived from the patient's medical history and the physical examination. The way the latter is performed will vary considerably among chiropractors, and will frequently be determined by the system to which the chiropractor subscribes. For example, a practitioner who subscribes to the method called applied kinesiology will have a set of specific physical tests spelled out by that method. There is also frequently widespread disagreement about these tests within chiropractic, as there is with applied kinesiology. Furthermore, the diagnosis in chiropractic retains its tentative nature in that the therapy and the response are used as ways of either confirming or revising the initial hunch.

In contrast, in modern medicine, diagnosis could be considered the climactic step in the treatment of disease. It is generally a routine procedure, it uses objective tests, can focus on all the systems of the body, and may involve numerous other functionaries. Where possible, it aims at a full differential diagnosis. In many ways, the great achievement of modern medicine is the advances made in diagnosis, and particularly in early diagnosis. Once the diagnosis is formed, the treatment procedure is also relatively standard. While there are many illnesses that are exceptions to this – that is, that do not lend themselves to a definitive diagnosis – the paradigm of medicine is to get them into this form. This is most clearly seen in the treatment of mental illness where, although definitive diagnosis of schizophrenia was historically not possible, it was treated as though this was the case. Behavioural abnormalities were interpreted as though they were a disordered pathology.

Explanation to the patient

Generally speaking, medicine uses a body of concepts and a language not accessible to the lay public. Much of medical education is spent mastering this language. Historically, this was reinforced by the use of Latin to ensure that the patient could not understand prescriptions written by the physician. Chiropractic, although dealing with the same biological complexity, has some distinct advantages. Since chiropractors do not prescribe drugs, they have little need to know the extensive pharmacology of the medical physician (although chiropractors do study pharmacology and must know some of the effects of drugs on the patient). Because they deal with functional pathology, they are able to use mechanical descriptions of the patient's problem and the physical treatment in ways readily understandable in a culture steeped in mechanical images. Modern society to a large extent understands the world mechanically, and technology is a major source of our metaphors. Combined with anatomical and neurological charts, small models of the spine and X-rays, the chiropractor also has highly visual means for explanations. Because chiropractic has been non-conventional, the chiropractor spends considerable time explaining (justifying) chiropractic itself, and this includes explanations of the philosophy of chiropractic. The latter is seldom part of a medical encounter. Since chiropractic involves, to a large degree, co-operative care, even in the sense of using the levers of the patient's body to give the manipulation, it is a form of care that requires 'recruitment' of the patient. This is seen most clearly in cervical manipulation where, without the patient relaxing and co-operating with the chiropractor, it is very difficult to complete the adjustment successfully. Last but not least, much of the chiropractic explanation is about the patient's lifestyle, providing an expanded opportunity for discussion and explanation. Whatever the cause, patients have a sense that they understand chiropractic in a way few report understanding medicine.

The treatment plan

As noted above, the climactic event in medicine for the physician is the diagnosis. Once this has been established, there is often a routine plan of treatment and, increasingly, a set of guidelines. To continue using our example of diabetes, in general practice once the diagnosis has been made and the type and stage of diabetes determined, there is a generally agreed standard of treatment to be followed. The patient will need to be monitored for complications and reactions to the treatment, but once the plan has been established the patient merely follows it. In the case of drugs, the patient receives the prescription, the pharmacist provides the drugs, and the patient takes them. So for much of medical care, the plan may be restricted to a single visit, and the patient's role is relatively passive and confined to compliance. This is reflected in the tremendous interest shown in medical care in the issue of compliance. Again there are clearly exceptions to this, but much of medicine in general practice follows this pattern, and therefore much of what the patients experience is this form of care. In one sense, this represents successful care in medicine. Where it fails, the patient must either be hospitalized or changed to a more aggressive form of treatment, and monitored more closely.

In chiropractic, the plan of treatment tends to be an elaborate procedure. It is seldom limited to one visit. The mean number of visits for low back pain is 14 and the median seven; for other problems it is nine visits with a median of four[6]. Furthermore, the plan is based on continuing assessment of the patient's functioning. For long-term chronic conditions, it may involve continuous care. The care is also provided at each step by the chiropractor, and virtually always involves the chiropractor doing something to the patient on each visit. In medicine, the continuing monitoring can be done by others. For example, where the patient's blood pressure must be monitored over a period, this can be carried out by the nurse, the nurse practitioner, the physicians' assistant, etc. In chiropractic, the plan of treatment is both an extension of the diagnosis itself and a

We have noted many times throughout this book that chiropractic is holistic, although the extent to which it is holistic is debatable. In the area of treatment this means that, as well as tending to the physical problem, the chiropractor will expand the care into areas such as exercise, nutrition, stress management, diet, posture and work habits. While much of this advice will simply concern such things as sleeping positions, for example, it can also involve a major lifestyle change, and requires patients to do things between the visits. These predominantly concern activities related to neuromusculoskeletal problems, such as stretching, exercising, applying ice or heat, altering how patients do things (like lifting) and correcting posture. Nutrition advice, stress management, relaxation techniques, vitamin supplements and weight loss are also reported by over 25 per cent of the patient population as being recommended by their chiropractors[6].

Evaluation of treatment

It is difficult to assess the importance of evaluation in medical care. For many of the conditions seen in general practice, the patient is diagnosed, a treatment is prescribed and, unless some complication occurs, there may be no further contact for this particular problem. Even where an evaluation does occur, it is carried out predominantly by the physician.

Evaluation is an integral part of the actual treatment in chiropractic. As noted earlier, there is highly pragmatic orientation in chiropractic care. Patients come to chiropractic because they fail to get results from other health-care providers, and they will remain with chiropractic only if they receive results. As a historically non-conventional provider, chiropractors faced the same challenge as all alternative providers. There is no cultural pressure or expectation for a person to go to a chiropractor. In the case of medicine, even where a person does not receive satisfactory results the cultural norm is that, on the next illness, the individual will invariably go to the medical physician. Even for those who have used chiropractic care in the past, 32 per cent will still go to the medical physician prior to the chiropractic for what would seem to be chiropractic-type complaints[7]. So firmly entrenched is medicine in our culture that, in a way not true for alternative health providers, getting results does not have the same importance. This is not to suggest that medicine does not get results, or that physicians do not care about getting results for their patients. It does suggest that the need to get results to survive in practice has characterized the chiropractic approach to treatment, in a way distinct from medicine.

Furthermore, the evaluation is immediate following an adjustment. This can occur in several ways. First, a patient may assess whether the pain has lessened. This may be assisted by the chiropractor using his hands to try and reproduce the pain in the musculature and soft tissues. Frequently the adjustment itself will relieve the tension and tenderness in these structures. Second, the patient and the provider may perform a functional analysis immediately after the adjustment. This occurs by the patient getting off the adjusting table and performing a range of motions to determine whether there has been any increase in the range of movement. Where the range has not improved, or not improved to the satisfaction of the chiropractor, the patient can be adjusted again. Third, each visit to a chiropractor begins anew with a physical evaluation, in which the chiropractor can reassess the improvement or lack of improvement since the last visit. Evaluation therefore plays a central role within chiropractic care, and tends to be a mutual affair. It is not unusual in a chiropractic office for patients to initiate and conduct the functional analysis themselves. This is frequently the case for patients such as those who are professional sports players, dancers or musicians – that is, those for whom the proper functioning of their physical structures is essential to their performance.

Termination of the case

In medicine, the extent to which a formal termination occurs varies considerably. It may terminate with the actual diagnosis itself. In many instances the patient follows the prescribed care and, if the particular ailment clears up, simply does not return. In these instances there is no ritual termination and, for the most part, the physician will not know when the termination of the care occurred. If the patient does not return, then the treatment is assumed to have been successful. For another group of patients, particularly those with serious illness or trauma requiring hospitalization, there will be a formal termination when the treatment is either judged to have been completed (as in surgery) or to have been successful (as in the treatment of pneumonia). In the case of long-term chronic conditions, there may never be a termination. The patient will have continuing care by the physician. For the final group of patients, those terminally ill or with serious trauma, termination occurs with death.

In chiropractic, termination may occur by the patient quitting the programme and simply failing to come again. The patient may also die. In the case of patients with chronic problems, there may never be a formal termination. However, for most patients termination of care tends to be a formal and negotiated affair. At the beginning of the treatment process the chiropractor usually tries to identify the type of improvement he or she will be trying to achieve, and a likely time frame in which it can be achieved. As noted previously, evaluation will help to fix when this is reached to the mutual satisfaction of the patient and the provider. Termination is almost as problematic in chiropractic as the initial visit, particularly for first-time patients. If it occurs too soon, apart from the fact that the patient may not receive the full benefit, there is also the risk of the patient feeling rejected as a patient. Since many chiropractic patients come to the chiropractor with their status having previously been challenged, this is problematic. If the chiropractor extends the treatment beyond what the patient feels is necessary, there is the risk of erring in the opposite direction and being viewed as practising for economic gain. Again, termination must be understood within the context of alternative care in our culture. Although medicine has frequently made the claim that the alternatives have no efficacy and involve the patient in lengthy and unnecessary care, this perspective totally ignores that if this were the case, and if the alternatives did not get results, they would have gone out of business well before now. Given that chiropractic patients are frequently well-educated[8], we can assume that they are not all gullible. Acceptable termination in chiropractic is therefore the key to whether a patient will return for some new problem in the future, and few chiropractors will remain in business very long if they do not build up such a clientele.

Conclusion

Chiropractic and medicine took quite different paths in the twentieth century. This is partly a reflection of their philosophical differences, but it is also a matter of opportunity and the development of their paradigms. Clearly, the scientific nature and development of the medical paradigm has spawned a whole range of therapies and opportunities for medicine. Furthermore, society has been willing so far to tolerate virtually any expansion of medicine, even while it may have serious moral objections to much of it – as seen in the current debates over embryo research, organ harvesting, genetic therapy, etc. Chiropractic, for its part, has been confined both legally and by patient choice to what at first seems a very narrow focus, that of the neuromusculoskeletal system. However, this apparently limited focus turns out to confer some decided advantages. First, these problems are seldom life-threatening or debilitating. Second, many of them have a natural history of recovery, others are responsive to care and some may be reversible. Third, this care can be achieved with the use of natural therapy. It is an area of practice, therefore, where the healer can daily experience the proof of the philosophy *vis medicatrix naturae*. Fourth, around these limited problems the chiropractors have been able to expand into wellness care. The end result is that the philosophy of chiropractic and the practice of chiropractic merge to create a health encounter that contrasts in significant ways to the medical health encounter. It is here that we find the secret of chiropractic's success, in the clinical art of chiropractic.

This success is no mean achievement. No single alternative profession has been singled out for opposition by medicine to the extent that chiropractic has. In the case of the American Medical Association, the objective was total annihilation. Furthermore, few (if any) professional groups have suffered the blatant bigotry and discrimination that chiropractors have been subjected to. While most of these are things of the past, they are not entirely absent even in the present. Chiropractic success, however, has never depended on acceptability by medicine, and although increasingly it is achieving that, its future will not depend on it. However, it will find increasing competition. The whole range of alternative health care is expanding and finding acceptance, and medicine itself is moving into integrative medicine – the combining of both medical and alternative care. Furthermore, as its own research paradigm expands, chiropractic may find one of two options occurring. On one hand, the research may substantiate the chiropractic role, as is already occurring with the efficacy of manipulation. This may then provide the basis for expansion into a broader-based practice. On the other hand, research may show that chiropractic has no efficacy outside a very narrow focus, and it will become more confined. While these issues may be fundamental in determining what insurance plans, governments and third party payers will cover in chiropractic services, none of this may matter if the patients decide for themselves that they will use chiropractic and pay for it out of pocket. The future of chiropractic, while it looks more promising than the past, is not without threats.

One thing that is clear from studying the history of chiropractic is that in one fundamental sense it is an alternative. Groups like chiropractic have kept alive an alternative philosophy of health. As outlined in this work, this has led to different conceptions of health care, the role of the healer, the role of the provider and, ultimately, the health encounter itself. To our earlier question, does philosophy make a difference, the answer given here is clearly that it does. Will it continue to do so in the future for chiropractic? This will largely depend on whether it does become genuine philosophy rather than dogma. For this to occur, chiropractors need to be better educated in philosophy, or to attract philosophers whose interest is in exploring chiropractic. They need to understand that philosophy involves subjecting all their concepts, including their most cherished ones such as the claim to treat the whole person, to critical scrutiny and debate. Chiropractic also needs to give up the insupportable claim that there is a chiropractic philosophy in favour of the claim that there can, and should, be a philosophy of chiropractic. Chiropractors need to draw on the general fields in philosophy in attempting to understand and articulate their vision for health care. They might also, by doing so, contribute to the general field of the philosophy of health.

References

[1] Coulter, I. D. (1983). Chiropractic and medical education. A contrast in models of health and illness. *J. Can. Chiropr. Ass.*, **27(4)**, 151–8.
[2] Cherkin, D., MacCormack, F. A. and Berg, A. D. (1988). Managing low back pain – a comparison of the beliefs and behaviors of family physicians and chiropractors. *West. J. Med.*, **149**, 476–80.
[3] Coulehan, J. L. (1985). Adjustment, the hands, and healing. *Cult. Med. Psychiatr.*, **9**, 353–82.
[4] Coulter, I. D. (1998). Efficacy and risks of chiropractic manipulation: what does the evidence suggest? *Integr. Med.*, **1(2)**, 61–6.

[5] Kelner, M., Hall, O. and Coulter, I. (1980). *Chiropractors: Do They Help.* Fitzhenry Whitesides.

[6] Coulter, I. D., Hays, R. D. and Danielson, C. D. (1996). The role of the chiropractor in the changing health-care system. From marginal to mainstream. *Res. Sociol. Health Care,* **13A,** 95–117.

[7] Coulter, I. D., Hurwitz, E. L., Adams, A. H. *et al.* (1998). Use of chiropractic services in North America: an empirical analysis. *Proc. Int. Conf. Spinal Manipul.,* pp. 3–4. Vancouver.

[8] Coulter, I. D. (1985). The chiropractic patient. A social profile. *J. Can. Chiropr. Ass.,* **29,** 25–8.

Epilogue

Two national surveys of adults in the United States[1,2] have shown not only extensive use of CAM by the population, but also that the numbers using CAM are increasing (from 33.8 per cent of the population in 1990 to 42.1 per cent in 1997). The estimated expenditure for this care was $21.2 billion in 1997, of which $12.2 billion were out-of-pocket expenditure. This exceeded the 1997 out-of-pocket expenditure for all US hospitalizations. Similar results have been shown for Australia[3] and for the use of CAM in Great Britain[4]. A recent Australian study[5] has shown that post-modern values of the population (values concerning nature, science, technology, health, authority, individual responsibility and consumerism) are the most predictive of attitudes towards alternative therapies. Dissatisfaction with medical outcomes accounted for only 4.2 per cent of the variance in attitudes to alternative therapies, and dissatisfaction with the health encounter 8 per cent, while post-modern values accounted for 27.8 per cent. Demographic variables did not have an impact on attitudes. Furthermore, it is not results with medical treatment but dissatisfaction with the way individuals are treated, the health encounter, that turns them away from mainstream care. The author[5] concludes that it is the emergence of a new philosophy that is the major explanation for the rise of alternative medicine. Furthermore, this philosophy is becoming more widespread and likely to contribute to even greater acceptability of alternative health care. In the chiropractic health encounter, the patient finds 'a logical set of beliefs which appeal to common sense, use scientific terminology, yet promote a natural, no-invasive, holistic approach rather than a medical approach'[6]. Both the patient and the chiropractor bring to the encounter a set of philosophical beliefs.

However, at this level we are using the word philosophy in a loose and undefined way. This work has also tried to show that the formal application of the concepts and methods of the discipline of philosophy will contribute to our understanding of alternative health care. As noted by Pellegrino[7], a philosophy *of* medicine *qua* medicine must focus on the clinical encounter. In this sense, what we have termed here the philosophy of chiropractic is simply a philosophy of medicine, where the latter is defined in its broader, generic sense and not just applied to allopathic medicine. While the analysis offered in this book is by necessity incomplete, it does illustrate the ways in which examining the alternative health providers helps us to understand concepts such as health, healing, health care, caring, illness and curing. As Pelligrino notes, medicine is concerned with the good of the patient which, in healing, means to make whole again. For the past 100 years, providers such as chiropractors have offered to the patient an alternative way in which that could happen. For the contemporary health care system, alternative medicine offers a different way of thinking about health and the nature of health care. We live in a time when, despite the incredible achievements of medical science and the vast resources put into the health care system, even advanced economic systems such as the United States have seen a steady rise in ill health throughout this century[8]. In this situation, a serious consideration of alternative health care would seem, *a priori*, not only appropriate but also necessary.

References

[1] Eisenberg, D. M., Kessler, R. C., Foster, C. *et al.* (1993). Unconventional medicine in the United States. *New Engl. J. Med.*, **328(4)**, 246–52.
[2] Eisenberg, D. M., Davis, R. B., Ettner, S. L. *et al.* (1998). Trends in alternative medicine use in the United States, 1990–1997. *JAMA*, **280(18)**, 1569–75.
[3] MacLenna, A. H., Wilson, D. H. and Taylor, A. W. (1996). Prevalence and cost of alternative medicine in Australia. *Lancet*, **347,** 569–73.
[4] Murray, J. and Shepherd, S. (1993). Alternative or additional medicine? An exploratory study in general practice. *Social Sci. Med.*, **37(8)**, 983–8.
[5] Siahpush, M. (1998). Post-modern values, dissatisfaction with conventional medicine and popularity of alternative therapies. *J. Sociol.*, **34(1),** 58–70.

[6] Coulehan, J. L. (1985). Chiropractic and the clinical art. *Social Sci. Med.*, **21(4)**, 383–90.

[7] Pellegrino, E. D. (1998). What the philosophy *of* medicine *is*. *Theor. Med. Bioeth.*, **19**, 315–36.

[8] Fulder, S. (1998). The basic concepts of alternative medicine and their impact on our views of health. *J. Alt. Compl. Med.*, **4(2)**, 147–58.

Index